Ace your emotions

A Useful Manual to Conquer Pessimism and Better Deal with Your Sentiment

Bill A. Jones

Ace your emotions

Table of contents

Ace your emotions

Ace your emotions

Disclaimer

Copyright © by Bill A. Jones 2023 Safeguarded by intellectual property regulation.
Before this record is duplicated or rehashed in any capacity,
the distributor's consent ought to be obtained. As needs be, the things
inside can nor be taken care of electronically, moved, nor kept
in an informational index. Neither somewhat nor full might the chronicle anytime at any point be
copied, inspected, faxed, or held without underwriting from the
distributor or creator.

Presentation

Individuals' emotion of dread toward dismissal particularly is a characteristic that shows frequently in day-to-day existence and makes life more troublesome in a ton of ways. Being acknowledged used to be a critical piece of actual endurance thus our minds are designed to look for it. Although being famous isn't as critical to remaining alive, people have areas of strength that should be preferred by others. Anxiety toward dismissal certainly isn't just about strict surrender yet numerous of all shapes and sizes. Emotion Irritated on the off chance that somebody snickers at you when you are being serious or doesn't giggle while you're making a joke. Disillusionment when others previously completed their food when you just showed up at the lunch table. Emotion Terrible when your words are misconstrued or over even the littlest basic remark. This multitude of circumstances feels perilous to the cerebrum, and it needs to gain from them to not confront them once more. To introduce one's best self, especially in proficient settings it is critical to know about this way of behaving and figure out how to recognize the genuine and fanciful danger

Expanding on these standards, the system-based models of Emotion Guideline depend on the verifiable suspicion that to forestall unfortunate effects, unwanted close-to-home states should be diminished through the choice and execution of modificatory techniques. Given this presumption, the models are adroitly unfit to represent hearty proof exhibiting those methodologies like mindfulness, acknowledgement, and resistance, which don't include decreases in that frame of mind among current and wanted states, in any case, leading to good emotional well-being. Considering this illustrative hole, it isn't to be expected that introductions of these models make no reference to such non-modificatory systems as significant parts of the procedure collection.

Another significant variable that influences our Emotions is dopamine. Dopamine is a synapse that assumes a huge part in compensating specific ways of behaving, and when it's delivered into the joy habitats of the mind it gives serious emotional prosperity like a high. Dopamine discharges for instance during activity or while betting, having intercourse or eating extraordinary food. This also integrates with endurance, the delight acquired from eating food propels an individual to search for it.Thinking emphatically isn't generally a simple assignment, yet it is surely connected to extraordinary advantages for the state of mind and well-being. Truly the sorts of contemplations you could have, influence your state of mind and might influence your future, positively or not. In that sense, "In this way, quite possibly of the main expertise you can dominate is your capacity to get a handle on your viewpoints and Emotions . This involves understanding what your Emotions are, how they work, and what reason they serve.

Section 1

Emotions and nature

Emotions are responses that people insight into in light of occasions or circumstances. The kind of Emotional individual not entirely set in stone by the situation that sets off the inclination. For example, an individual encounters euphoria when they get uplifting news. Individuals encounter dread when they are compromised.

Emotions affect our regular routines. We go with choices given whether we are cheerful, furious, miserable, exhausted, or disappointed. We pick exercises and side interests in light of the Emotions they prompt. Understanding Emotions can assist us with exploring existence effortlessly and dependably.

While specialists accept that various essential general Emotions are capable by individuals all around the world paying little mind to foundation or culture, scientists additionally accept that encountering emotions can be exceptionally subjective.5 Think about outrage, for instance. Is all outrage something very similar? Your own experience could go from gentle inconvenience to blinding fury.

While we have expansive marks for Emotions , for example, "irate," "miserable," or "cheerful," your insight of these Emotions might be considerably more multi-layered, thus abstract

We likewise don't necessarily encounter unadulterated types of every inclination. Blended Emotions over various occasions or circumstances in our lives are normal. When confronted with beginning a new position, you could feel both invigorated and anxious. Getting hitched or having a kid may be set apart by a wide assortment of Emotions going from delight to tension. These Emotions could happen at the same time, or you could feel them consistently.

Emotions are mental states welcomed by neurophysiological changes, differently connected with considerations, sentiments, conduct reactions, and a level of delight or disappointment. There is right now no logical agreement on a definition. feeling, a complicated encounter of cognizance, substantial sensation, and conduct that mirrors the individual meaning of a thing, an occasion, or a province of affairs. The assortment and intricacy of Emotions

"Emotions ," composed Aristotle (384-322 BCE), "are those sentiments that so change men as to influence their decisions, and that are additionally gone to by agony or delight. Such are an outrage, pity, dread and so forth, with their contrary energies." Emotion is for sure a heterogeneous class that includes a wide assortment of significant mental peculiarities. A few Emotions are unmistakable, to the extent that they concern a specific individual, item, or circumstance. Others, like pain, euphoria, or discouragement, are exceptionally broad. A few Emotions are extremely concise and scarcely cognizant, like an unexpected flush of humiliation or an explosion of outrage. Others, like dependable love or stewing hatred, are extended, enduring hours, months, or even years (in which case they can turn into a tough component of a singular character). An inclination might have articulated actual backups, like a look, or it could be imperceptible to onlookers. An inclination might include cognizant experience and reflection, as when one "flounders" in it, or it might pass essentially inconspicuously and unacknowledged by the

Ace your emotions

subject. An inclination might be significant, as it is fundamental for one's actual endurance or psychological well-being, or it could be minor or broken. An inclination might be socially suitable or improper. It might try and be socially mandatory — e.g., Emotionregret in the wake of perpetrating wrongdoing or Emotionpain at a memorial service.

As needs be, there is a colossal scope of Emotions , and, surprisingly, inside the equivalent "Emotion Families" there is extensive variety. Frenzy and dread, for instance, are many times remembered to be fellow Emotions , yet there is a tremendous contrast between the frenzy that is appeared in a nonsensical trepidation or a fear and a savvy dread — like the emotional dread toward atomic conflict — which requires a fair plan of data and examination. Dread and awfulness, two other fellow Emotions , are by and by unmistakable from dread. Or on the other hand, consider the gigantic group of threatening Emotions similar to outrage: rage, wrath, disdain, hatred, disdain, despising, and contempt, to give some examples. Those Emotions are strangely divergent in their design and their suitable settings, as are individuals from the "self-basic family," which incorporates disgrace, shame, culpability, regret, and lament. The extraordinary assortment and wealth of Emotions propose that the class of emotion may not be a solitary class of mental peculiarities but rather a huge group of inexactly related mental states and cycles.

For effortlessness, analysts and laypeople the same frequently partition the Emotions into those that are "good" and those that are "pessimistic." However, the intricacy of Emotions delivers such restrictions. Even though adoration and disdain, for instance, are frequently considered perfect inverses, they

Ace your emotions

must regularly exist together not as contrary energies but rather as supplements. Additionally, love is frequently excruciating and horrendous, and scorn, now and again, can be positive. Yet, an inclination like displeasure, another purported pessimistic inclination, shows the uselessness of such a characterization. Outrage is without a doubt a gloomy inclination coordinated toward someone else, yet it tends to be illuminating for the irate individual, and, in the suitable setting — a setting wherein one should be furious — it can helpfully affect what is happening or a relationship. In this way, the women's activist development moved forward when ladies understood that they reserved a privilege to be irate and much to be furious about. It very well might be, as Aristotle noticed, that Emotions are joined by delight or agony, however, they are excessively mind-boggling and frequently too unpretentious to be in any way grouped on that premise alone.

feeling

The investigation of Emotions was long the territory of morals. Emotions were fundamental to Aristotle's morals of prudence and a vital part of the middle age Scholastics' anxiety with indecencies, temperances, and sin. For Aristotle, having the perfect proportion of the right emotion in the right conditions is the way to a prudent way of behaving. St. Thomas Aquinas (c. 1224-74) recognized "higher" and "lower" Emotions , the previous exemplified with conviction and love, the last option by outrage and jealousy. Albeit moral pondering Emotions has forever been worried about profound limits and abnormalities, as in psychopathology and franticness, those peculiarities have never been the essential justification for interest in the Emotions . As Aristotle and the middle age moralists saw very well, Emotions are crucial for a solid human life, and it is thus that their breakdown is so serious.

The appropriate turn of events and working of Emotions permit individuals to live well and be content. Love, regard, and sympathy, for instance, are the fundamental close-to-home elements of relational relations and concerns. Emotions persuade moral (as well as shameless) conduct, and they assume a fundamental part in imagination and logical interest. For some individuals, Emotions are animated and incited by excellence in human expression and nature, and there is no tasteful reasonableness without feeling. Emotions as well as the actual faculties shape the fundamental cycles of discernment and memory and impact the manners by which individuals imagine and decipher their general surroundings (clinicians have long known that what one notices and recalls relies by and large upon what one thinks often about). While certain Emotions can gain out of influence and harm one's very own prosperity and social connections, most Emotions are practical and versatile. By the by, the way that such countless individuals experience the ill effects of "profound issues" during their lives makes figuring out the pathology of Emotions a standing social concern.

Ace your emotions

The design of Emotions

Emotions have been concentrated on in a few logical disciplines — e.g., science, brain research, neuroscience, psychiatry, human studies, and social science — as well as in business the executives, publicizing, and correspondences. Accordingly, unmistakable points of view on emotion have arisen, proper to the intricacy and assortment of the actual Emotions . It is significant, be that as it may, to take those alternate points of view not as seriously but rather as corresponding, each possibly yielding knowledge into what might be known as the unique "structures" of Emotions . To say that Emotions have structures is to dismiss the view that they are simply formless "sentiments" or that they have no structure, rationale, or discernment. Going against the norm, Emotions are organized in more than one way:

by their fundamental nervous system science, by the decisions and assessments that go into them, by the way of behaving that communicates or shows them, and by the bigger social settings in which they happen. Hence, it could be said that an inclination is a"coordinated neuro-physiological-conduct evaluative-experiential-social peculiarity." Various Emotions will show such designs to various degrees and in various ways, contingent upon the particular inclination, its sort, and the conditions.

 the designs of the various Emotions will be viewed under three headings (however it ought to be borne as a top priority that the designs of any inclination are constantly incorporated into a natural entirety):

(1) actual designs, including a plain way of behaving, nervous system science, and physiology

Ace your emotions

(2) experiential designs, or how an inclination is capable by the subject

(3) social designs, including social causes and conditions, the social significance and capability of profound articulations, the social impacts of close to home way of behaving, the political circumstances and results of close to home way of behaving, and the moral contemplations that decide the nature and propriety of Emotions .

Actual designs of feeling

During the main portion of the twentieth hundred years, individuals from the mental school of behaviourism endeavoured to concentrate on mental peculiarities stringently concerning their freely detectable circumstances and results. As per behaviourists, any logical record of Emotions should be restricted to a depiction of the discernible conditions that summon Emotions (the "upgrade") and the noticeable actual changes and conduct that outcome from them (the "reaction"), including a particular verbal way of behaving. Although behaviourism is not generally viewed as a reasonable methodology, it ought to be noted exactly how much the component of the openly recognizable envelops. The boost and reaction circumstances incorporate not just the actual environmental elements of individuals encountering the inclination and any development, signal, or sound they make yet additionally their neurological, neurochemical, and physiological states — including, for instance, chemical levels and varieties in the action of the autonomic sensory system, which controls and manages inside organs.

The neurobiology of feeling

Ace your emotions

Before the coming of behaviourism, when the study of nervous system science was still in its earliest stages, the American scholar and analyst William James (1842-1910) brought a portion of the elements together in his hypothesis of feeling, which he set out in his central review The Standards of Brain research (1890). In about a couple of dozen pages, James referred to a wide assortment of physiological changes engaged with certain Emotions : autonomic sensory system movement (dashing heart, enlargement of the veins, tightening of the bladder and guts, compulsory changes in breathing, and "something in the pharynx that urges either a swallow, a getting free from the throat, or a slight hack"), trademark "close to home" cerebrum processes, "apprehensive expectations," and obvious actual articulations and activities — shudder, sobbing, running, and striking. For James, such Emotions are actual impressions that go with specific physiological changes that themselves are achieved by some "disturbing" insight. Likewise, in a well-known recommendation, he encouraged the people who wished to work on their close-to-home state to "smooth the forehead, light up the eye, contract the dorsal as opposed to the ventral part of the casing, and talk in a significant key, and pass the inclination, a complicated encounter of cognizance, substantial sensation, and conduct that mirrors the individual meaning of a thing, an occasion, or a situation.

Research has since recognized the substantial changes considered by James. Autonomic sensory system movement, which is once in a while taken to be the centre of James' hypothesis, is unmistakable from deliberate muscle action. Contemporary nervous system science has come to zero in significantly more on mind movement accordingly and to regard any remaining substantial changes as stringently auxiliary. Neuroscientific research has shown not just that Emotions have their beginnings in brain activity in the cerebrum yet that various Emotions show altogether different examples of brain action. The centre of close-to-home mind action is by all accounts the limbic forebrain: the thalamus, the nerve centre, the reticular arrangement, and the amygdala, which are all subcortical (beneath the cerebral cortex). The nerve centre has significant connections to joy and hopelessness, while the reticular arrangement might have a significant connection to despondency. The American neuroscientist Joseph E. LeDoux has shown that the hear-able excitement of dread includes the transmission of sound signs through the hear-able pathway to the thalamus (which transfers data) and afterwards to the dorsal amygdala (which assesses data). Such exploration recommends that emotion that is initiated via the thalamus-amygdala pathway results from evaluative handling that is quick, negligible, and programmed. In any case, emotion may likewise be enacted through a transfer of data from the thalamus to the neocortex (the external piece of the cerebral cortex), and this circuit is the brain's reason for the mental examination and assessment of occasions. In this way, there are two brain processes associated with the actuation of Emotions : cortical and subcortical. The initiation of emotion through the thalamus-amygdala pathway makes sense of how babies and extremely small kids answer genuinely to agony and why grown-ups have major areas of strength for expressing and causing profound decisions before they have any cognizant acknowledgement of doing as such. Individuals frequently

Ace your emotions

experience emotion before they structure explanations behind having the Emotions they do.

The two halves of the globe of the mind are connected contrastingly to profound cycles. The right half of the globe might be more capable than the left at separating between close-to-home articulations. Additionally, it has been contended that the right side of the equator might be more associated with handling gloomy Emotions and the left half of the globe more engaged with handling good Emotions . Individuals who are restless, irate, or discouraged show expanded movement in the amygdala and the right prefrontal cortex. Individuals Emotiongood show expanded action in the left prefrontal

cortex, while the amygdala and the right prefrontal cortex stay calm. A great many people experience the two kinds of temperaments and Emotions , however, people likewise appear to have a pretty much fixed natural inclination to be content or to be restless. Indeed, even after favourable luck or horrible luck, individuals ultimately will quite often get back to their run-of-the-mill everyday mindsets. (There is some proof, notwithstanding, that activities like reflection can move a normal state of mind toward the positive.) Throughout the long term, there have been different speculations about precisely where the brain bases of Emotionlie. Yet, the most conceivable speculations demand that mind capabilities overall include complex collaborations between various parts; subsequently, the mission for the "middle" of Emotionmight be off track

The conduct articulation of Emotionlikewise incorporates cognizant and oblivious motions, stances and peculiarities, and a clear way of behaving that can be either unconstrained or conscious. One could wonder whether or not to consider the purposeful way of behaving an "articulation" because of the mediating cognizant movement it includes. One could talk rather than a such way of behaving as being "out of" the inclination (as in, "he carried on of outrage"). However, the distinction between the two cases is much of the time extremely slight. Carrying on of outrage might be quick, as on account of an unconstrained affront, or it could be extended or deferred. It could be communicated in a progression of reformatory activities that happen for months or years or in vindictive demonstrations that follow the inciting event and the displeasure by a similarly extensive timeframe. Yet, even the quick articulation of emotional obvious activity might be (and typically is) extended in time and not just flitting. Running from risk in dread might happen however long it needs to (as long as the danger is obvious). The declaration of significant love, many individuals would agree, happens for a lifetime, however, it might likewise comprise quite a few both unconstrained and intentional demonstrations and motions.

Verbal articulations are specifically compelling. They can be unconstrained and prompt, just like the hoots and cheers of avid supporters, however, they can be more smooth, articulate, and intentional. A memorial service discourse might be sincere and expressive of the emotion of pain; a statement of regret can likewise be genuine and expressive of the Emotions of disgrace and regret. What's more, obviously the recitation of an affection sonnet can act as a broad "I love you."Experiential designs of feeling

James presented his hypothesis of Emotions with a significant capability: "I ought to express above all else that the main Emotions I propose explicitly to consider here are those that have an unmistakable substantial articulation." Even though there are Emotions that have no such articulation, James demanded that all Emotions have a psychological or cognizant aspect.

The starting reason for feeling, as per James, is an insight. James didn't take insight to be a constituent of feeling, yet he perceived its significance. To place the matter such that he didn't, James perceived that an inclination should be "tied in with" something. It isn't simply an inclination because of a physiological unsettling influence. Accordingly, James implied deliberateness, the component of a few mental cycles in the temperance of which they are basically about or coordinated toward an item. Numerous scholars following James have modified his examination by including insight and with it deliberateness, as a fundamental piece of feeling. For sure, a few scholars have guaranteed that an inclination is only an extraordinary sort of insight. The idea of profound experience, as needs be, has been extensively improved to incorporate not just actual vibes of what is happening in one's body yet in addition perceptual encounters of what is happening in the world. In the investigation of feeling, that point of view is a personal point of view, "hued" by the different Emotions as well as by the one-of-a-kind point of view of the subject. In any case, the normal similitude of variety does

Profound experience likewise incorporates joy and torment, as Aristotle demanded, however seldom as detached sentiments. More regularly, various parts of an inclination are pleasurable or excruciating, as considerations or recollections might be pleasurable or agonizing. The inclination as such might be pleasurable or excruciating (e.g., pride or regret), thus may one's affirmation of the way that one has a specific inclination (charmed to be infatuated once more, annoyed with oneself for blowing up or desirous). In any case, once more, close to home matters are not generally so clear. It is normal to have "blended Emotions ," when the countercurrents of joy and torment make it hard to choose a solitary perspective.

Social designs of feeling

Even though Darwin felt that close to home articulations are because of "the constitution of the sensory system" and assume a part in variation and endurance, he accepted that others fill an alternate need: the correspondence of emotion to other people. For sure, the universality and consistency of looks of emotion would be difficult to understand if it were not for the way that they convey a singular's Emotions to different individuals from his gathering or species. By grinning one demonstrates benevolence and maybe the absence of purpose to hurt; by scowling one conveys the inverse. The close-to-home demeanours that are so obvious in the face and body act as the primary method for correspondence between a mother and her baby. As Darwin noted, "We promptly see compassion in others by their appearance; our sufferings are accordingly moderated. We giggle together and our shared pleasantness increments and reinforces our pleasure." The social part of the feeling, likewise, is most clear in broad daylight presentations of feeling, which straightforwardly influence the way of behaving of others. In any case, this perspective incorporates substantially more than correspondence. The social designs of emotion comprise the manners by which the bigger social setting decides an inclination's causes, content, methods of articulation, and importance. Indeed, even the fundamental Emotions , which are for the most part expected to have a neurological centre, are moulded generally by friendly variables.

Social setting decides the reasons for Emotions from a conspicuous perspective: various conditions incite various Emotions in various societies. A Vodou (Voodoo) revile, for instance, produces fear in one society but just bemusement in another. A spouse who sees his significant other in the organization of another man becomes desirous in one society but might be unconcerned in another. All Emotions include perception, and all are impacted by virtues and evaluative ideas, many (while perhaps not) of which are scholarly. The ideas of good and bad, suitable and improper and their legitimate application are learned in the particular conditions of each gathering or society

Emotions are dependent upon social moulding in their methods of articulation as in many articulations, maybe even those that are pretty much designed, are dependent upon the neighbourhood "show rules," which oversee which Emotions and which articulations are proper in which conditions. An outflow of outrage is completely unseemly in most open conditions in Japan, yet it is very not out of the ordinary at a metropolitan convergence in the US. The social significance of an inclination is additionally (and) still up in the air. In Tahiti outrage is viewed as very perilous and is even defamed; in the Mediterranean it is in many cases an indication of virility, recommending exemplary nature. It is not necessarily the case that the social impacts on emotion are restricted to their social translations. The actual Emotions are comprised, to some degree, of such understandings. The socially comprised piece of an inclination might be more modest in fundamental Emotions than in intellectually rich Emotions like moral resentment and heartfelt love, yet culture as well as science, social contrasts as well as individual contrasts, figure

Ace your emotions

out what Emotions there are and whether, where, and when having them is suitable.

Emotions and sanity

The way that Emotions include conduct, contemplations, and culture brings up the issue of whether or how much Emotions are objective. For logicians like Plato (c. 428-c. 348 BCE) and David Hume (1711-76), who considered emotion and reasonableness as clashing contrary energies, such an inquiry was unseemly all along. In any case, conduct and considerations can be objective or silly, and culture forces its principles of reasonableness. To that degree, at any rate, close-to-home articulations and contemplations can be decided by such norms. Out of resentment, individuals frequently act and think unreasonably. In any case, what is now and again underscored is that outrage can bring about conduct and considerations that are very levelheaded, as in they are decisively fruitful in articulating or directing the emotion into useful activity. The considerations that one has out of resentment may likewise be precise and clever — e.g., recalling past insults and an example of a hostile way of behaving. What's more, culture, forces its standards for concluding which articulations and considerations are judicious, as well as which Emotions having in which circumstances is sane. To be desirous of specific societies and specific conditions might be completely suitable and in this manner reasonable. In any case, in different societies or different conditions, envy is unseemly and along these lines unreasonable.

An inclination can likewise be objective or nonsensical in two additional particulars detects:

(1) it very well may be pretty much exactly in the discernment or comprehension of the circumstance it includes

(2) it tends to be pretty much justified in its assessment of the circumstance. An illustration of (1) is: Joel resents denial for offering something hostile when Jones said nothing of the sort and there is not a great explanation to believe that he did. An illustration of (2) is: Joel resents denial for offering something hostile, yet, as a matter of fact, what Jones said was not hostile since it was not deliberate or because it was an exact and helpful analysis of Smith, for which Smith ought not to be outraged or irate. In the main model, the outrage is silly since it depends on deception about the circumstance; in the subsequent, it is nonsensical because it includes an out-of-line or uncalled-for assessment.

In one more sense, Emotions can be level headed to the extent that they are utilitarian. It has become something of a maxim in contemporary brain science that Emotions have developed alongside people and are thus the result of the normal determination. It doesn't follow, notwithstanding, that a specific inclination was separately chosen for, or that Emotions serve, the capabilities that might have made them important previously. Outrage might have been a valuable upgrade of hostility in ancient times, however, it very well may be harmful or largely useless in a cutting-edge metropolitan climate. Additionally, Emotions (or specific Emotions) likely could be the results of other developed qualities. All things considered when in doubt, Emotions do

Ace your emotions

assume a significant part in individuals' private and public activities. To be sure, Hume demanded that explanation without anyone else giving no inspiration for a moral way of behaving; just Emotions can do that. Current neuroscience has reached a lot of similar ends.

However, emotions can be objective as in they can be utilised to accomplish specific fundamental human objectives and desires. Lashing out might be a significant stage in rousing oneself to confront hindrances and defeat them. Falling head over heels might be a significant stage in fostering the ability to shape and keep up with personal connections. All the while, blowing up at one's supervisor might be completely justified yet at the same time unreasonable to the extent that it baffles one's vocational objectives. A Buddhist priest might be completely legitimate in being envious of an individual priest, yet his desire is all things considered nonsensical to the extent that it is contradictory with his origination of himself as a Buddhist. In this sense, Emotions give both the substance of a decent life and its closures. Along these lines, the French existentialist rationalist Jean-Paul Sartre (1905-80) contended that Emotions are techniques. Individuals use them to control others and, more significantly, to move into perspectives and acting that suit their objectives and their mental self-view.

Since Emotions are an item of culture as well as of one's way of behaving and perspectives over the long run, one is somewhat answerable to them. Emotions can be deliberately evolved or deterred via preparing oneself to respond pretty much genuinely — or with a greater amount of one sort of emotion and less of another — in specific conditions. For Aristotle, this sort of preparation is essential for the most common way of developing a decent upright person oneself.

Ace your emotions

Having the right Emotions in the perfect sums and the right conditions, as he contended, is the substance of temperance and the way to human

Physiological Reaction

Assuming you've at any point felt your stomach stagger from tension or your heart touch with dread, then you understand that Emotions additionally cause solid physiological responses

A large number of the physiological reactions you experience during an inclination, for example, sweat-soaked palms or a dashing heartbeat, are directed by the thoughtful sensory system, a part of the autonomic sensory system

The autonomic sensory system controls compulsory body reactions, for example, bloodstream and assimilation. The thoughtful sensory system is accused of controlling the body's survival responses. While confronting a danger, these reactions naturally set up your body to escape from risk or face the danger head-on

While early investigations of the physiology of Emotionwould in general zero in on these autonomic reactions, later examination plays designated the mind's part in Emotions .

Cerebrum checks have shown that the amygdala, a piece of the limbic framework, assumes a significant part in Emotion and dread specifically

The actual amygdala is a minuscule, almond-moulded structure that has been connected to inspirational states like yearning and thirst as well as memory and feeling. Specialists have utilised cerebrum imaging to show that when individuals are shown compromising pictures, the amygdala becomes enacted. Harm to the amygdala has additionally been displayed to impede the apprehension reaction

The 6 Sorts of Essential Emotions and Their Impact on the Human Way of behaving

Medicinally checked on by Steven Gans, MD

There is a wide range of sorts of Emotions that impact how we live and collaborate with others. On occasion, it might appear as though we are controlled by these Emotions . Our decisions, the moves we make, and the discernments we have are completely affected by the Emotions we are encountering out of the blue.

Analysts have likewise attempted to distinguish the various kinds of Emotions that individuals experience. One or two hypotheses have arisen to classify and make sense of the Emotions that individuals feel.

Consolidating Emotions

Clinician Robert Plutchik set forth a "wheel of Emotions " that worked something like the variety wheel. Emotions can be joined to shape various sentiments, similar to varieties that can be blended to make different shades.

As per this hypothesis, the more fundamental Emotions act something like structure blocks. More complicated, once in a while blended Emotions , are blendings of these more essential ones. For instance, fundamental Emotions , for example, euphoria and trust can be consolidated to make love.

A recent report proposes that there are undeniably more fundamental Emotions than beforehand believed.1 In the review distributed in Procedures of Public Foundation of Sciences, scientists distinguished 27 distinct classifications of feeling.

As opposed to being completely particular, in any case, the specialists found that individuals experience these Emotions along a slope.

Firstly, Let's investigate a portion of the fundamental sorts of Emotions and investigate the effect they have on the human way of behaving.

• Bliss

Of the multitude of various sorts of Emotions , joy will in general be the one that individuals take a stab at the most. Bliss is much of the time characterised as a wonderful close-to-home expression that is portrayed by sensations of happiness, delight, satisfaction, fulfilment, and prosperity.

Research on satisfaction has expanded essentially since the 1960s inside various disciplines, including the part of brain science known as sure brain science. This sort of Emotion at times communicated through.Bliss has been connected to various results including expanded life span and expanded conjugal satisfaction.On the other hand, despondency has been connected to an assortment of chronic weakness results.

•Manner of speaking

Ace your emotions

a cheery, wonderful approach to talking

While satisfaction is viewed as one of the fundamental human Emotions , the things we think will make bliss will generally be vigorously impacted by culture. For instance, mainstream society impacts will quite often underline that achieving specific things like purchasing a home or having lucrative work will bring about satisfaction.

The real factors of what add to satisfaction are many times considerably more mind-boggling and all the more exceptionally individualized.Individuals have long accepted that bliss and well-being were associated, and research has upheld the possibility that joy can assume a part in both physical and emotional well-being.

Stress, tension, despondency, and dejection, for instance, have been connected to things like brought down insusceptibility, expanded irritation, and diminished future.

•Bitterness

Bitterness is one more kind of Emotion Frequently characterised as a transient profound state described by sensations of frustration, distress, sadness, lack of engagement, and a hosed mindset.

Like different Emotions , trouble is something that all individuals experience every once in a while. Now and again, individuals can encounter drawn-out and serious times of misery that can transform into wretchedness. Bitterness can be communicated in various ways including:

Crying

Hosed temperament

Dormancy

Ace your emotions

Quietness

Withdrawal from others

The sort and seriousness of misery can fluctuate contingent on the underlying driver, and how individuals adapt to such sentiments can likewise vary.

Trouble can frequently lead individuals to participate in ways of dealing with hardship or stress, for example, staying away from others, self-curing, and ruminating on bad considerations. Such ways of behaving can really fuel sensations of misery and draw out the span of the inclination.

•Dread

Dread is a strong emotion that can likewise assume a significant part in endurance. At the point when you face some kind of risk and experience dread, you go through what is known as the survival reaction.

Your muscles become tense, your pulse and breath increment and your brain wakes up, preparing your body for one or the other run from the risk or stand and fight.

This reaction guarantees that you are ready to manage dangers in your current circumstance successfully. Articulations of this kind of Emotion Can include:

Physiological responses like quick breathing and heartbeat.

Obviously, not every person encounters dread similarly. Certain individuals might be more delicate to fear and certain circumstances or articles might be bound to set off this inclination.

Dread is the personal reaction to a prompt danger. We can likewise foster a comparable response to expected dangers or even our considerations about possible risks, and this is our thought process of nervousness. Social tension, for instance, includes an expected emotion of dread toward social circumstances.

Certain individuals, then again, really search out dread-inciting circumstances. Outrageous games and different rashes can be dread prompting, however, certain individuals appear to flourish and try and appreciate such sentiments.

Rehashed openness to a trepidation item or circumstance can prompt commonality and acclimation, which can lessen sensations of dread and nervousness.

This is the thought behind openness treatment, where individuals are steadily presented with the things that terrify them in a controlled and safe way. Ultimately, sensations of dread start to diminish.

•Disdain

Disdain is one more of the first six fundamental Emotions portrayed by Eckman. Nausea can be shown in various ways including:

Non-verbal communication: getting some distance from the object of disdain

Actual responses: like heaving or spewing

Looks, for example, wrinkling the nose and twisting the upper lip

This emotion of repugnance can begin from various things, including a disagreeable taste, sight, or smell. Specialists accept that this emotion developed as a response to food sources that may be destructive or lethal. At the point when individuals smell or taste food varieties that have turned sour, for instance, disdain is a normal response.

Unfortunate cleanliness, disease, blood, decay, and demise can likewise set off a repugnance reaction. This might be the

Ace your emotions

body's approach to keeping away from things that might convey communicable infections.

Individuals can likewise encounter moral nausea when they notice others participating in ways of behaving that they view as disagreeable, corrupt, or evil.

•Outrage

Outrage can be an especially strong inclination described by sensations of aggression, tumult, disappointment, and threat towards others. Like trepidation, outrage can have an impact on your body's survival reaction.

At the point when a danger produces sensations of outrage, you might be leaned to fight off the risk and safeguard yourself. Outrage is frequently shown through:

Looks:

for example, grimacing or glaring

Non-verbal communication:

like taking areas of strength for an or dismissing

Manner of speaking, for example, talking bluntly or hollering

Physiological reactions:

like perspiring or becoming red

Forceful ways of behaving:

 like hitting, kicking, or tossing objects

While outrage is much of the time considered a pessimistic inclination, it can some of the time be great. It tends to be useful in explaining your necessities in a relationship, and it can likewise spur you to make a move and find answers for things that are irritating you.

Outrage can turn into an issue, nonetheless, when unnecessary or communicated in manners that are unfortunate, risky, or

Ace your emotions

unsafe to other people. Uncontrolled indignation can rapidly go to animosity, misuse, or brutality.

Outrage Issues:

Step through the Examination

This sort of emotion can have both mental and actual outcomes. Uncontrolled outrage can go with it hard to settle on judicious decisions and could affect your actual well-being. Outrage has been connected to coronary heart sicknesses and diabetes. It has additionally been connected to ways of behaving that act as well-being dangers such as forceful driving, liquor utilisation, and smoking.

•Shock

Shock is another of the six fundamental sorts of human Emotions initially portrayed by Eckman. Shock is typically very short and is portrayed by a physiological frightened reaction following something surprising.

This kind of emotion can be good, pessimistic, or unbiased. An unsavoury shock, for instance, could include somebody leaping out from behind a tree and terrifying you as you stroll to your vehicle around evening time.

An illustration of a wonderful little treat would get back to find that your dearest companions have accumulated praise your birthday. Shock is frequently portrayed by:

Looks:

 like raising the temples, enlarging the eyes, and opening the mouth

Actual reactions: like bouncing back

Verbal responses: like hollering, shouting, or wheezing

Shock is one more sort of Emotion that can set off the survival reaction. When frightened, individuals might encounter an

Ace your emotions

explosion of adrenaline that readies the body to one or the other battle or escape.

Shock can significantly affect the human way of behaving. For instance, research has shown that individuals will more often than not lopsidedly notice astonishing occasions.

For this reason, astounding and surprising occasions in the news will generally hang out in memory more than others. Research has additionally observed that individuals will generally be more influenced by amazing contentions and advance more from astonishing data.

Different Kinds of Emotions

The six fundamental Emotions portrayed by Eckman are only a piece of a wide range of sorts of Emotions that individuals are fit for encountering. Eckman's hypothesis recommends that these central Emotions are general all through societies from one side of the planet to the other.

Be that as it may, different hypotheses and new explorations keep on investigating the various kinds of Emotions and how they are characterised. Eckman later added various Emotions to his rundown however proposed that dissimilar to his unique six Emotions , not these could essentially be encoded through looks. A portion of the Emotions he later recognized included:

Entertainment
Scorn
Satisfaction

Ace your emotions

Shame
Energy
Responsibility
Pride in accomplishment
Help
Fulfilment
Disgrace

Different Hypotheses of Feeling

Likewise, with numerous ideas in brain science, not all scholars settle on the most proficient method to arrange Emotions or what the essential Emotions are. While Eckman's hypothesis is one of the most incredibly known, different scholars have proposed their thoughts regarding what Emotions make up the centre of the human experience.

For instance, a few specialists have recommended that there are just a few fundamental Emotions . Others have recommended that Emotions exist in something of an ordered progression. Essential Emotions like love, delight, shock, outrage, and bitterness can then be additionally separated into auxiliary Emotions . Love, for instance, comprises optional Emotions , such as fondness and yearning.

These optional Emotions could then be separated even further into what is known as tertiary Emotions . The auxiliary emotion of friendship incorporates tertiary Emotions , like prefer, mindfulness, empathy, and delicacy.

A later report recommends that there are no less than 27 particular Emotions , which are all profoundly interconnected. All in all, Emotions are not states that happen in seclusion. All things considered, the review recommends that there are

angles of Emotion and that these various sentiments are
profoundly interrelated

<h1 style="text-align:center">Section 2</h1>

The most effective method to Comprehend and Communicate your Emotions

Human Emotions advanced with the goal that we can answer rapidly to crucial circumstances.

All things considered, while dread might keep us from acting in a 'daily existence restricting' way, outrage can drive us to safeguard ourselves or those nearest to us. While proof proposes a few Emotions are general, there is a nobody-size-fits-all close-to-home equilibrium that suits each culture or all people.

We ought to stay mindful and try not to view clients who might vary genuinely from ourselves as waiting to be fixed. Be that as it may, we as a whole advantage of a better comprehension of our Emotions and what they mean for our way of behaving, particularly when they conflict with our every day and long-lasting goals. how to comprehend and communicate your Emotions

Understanding sentiments and Emotions can be a troublesome excursion, in any event, when you know how to make it happen.

The Voice Of Outrage

During outrage you could understand that your heart is thumping quicker than expected, you're breathing quicker and perhaps shaking a tad. Your face and neck might feel hot and your clenched hands could grasp. At the point when we

Ace your emotions

become upset it's normal as far as we're concerned to need to shout, toss things, and even attack the other individual.

You might encounter considerations, for example, "I can't stand him" or "I can't completely accept that she did that"; "This is absurd" or "This is ridiculous!"; overwhelming inclinations of aggression; the motivation to fault others for your concerns; trouble concentrating, and additionally contemplations about vengeance.

Outrage is an extreme inclination or emotion that can be set off by a pessimistic occasion or connection. Outrage advises you to make a move of some kind or another — positive or negative. It can prompt animosity since your body is preparing itself for an actual counter of some kind.

Outrage can let us know that something is off-base and needs consideration. Outrage may likewise flag that something feels unjustifiable for instance, you could feel furious assuming that you're ignored for advancement at work notwithstanding the way that you have the best numbers in the workplace.

You might have to define suitable limits or figure out how to communicate outrage in manners that don't hurt yourself as well as other people, like figuring out how to say "no" or getting some margin to chill off. Assuming you battle with outrage, find the opportunity to look into accusing, disgracing, and controlling explanations. Give a valiant effort to convey in a solid manner, in any event, when it seems like displeasure is outwitting you. Outrage can be something to be thankful for assuming we allowed it to assist with persuading us to change our conditions or ways of behaving to improve things

The Voice Of Dread

While you're Emotionterrified, your heart could pulsate quickly and hard, you could start to perspire a tad, feel winded

Ace your emotions

or hyperventilate. You might become tense all through your entire body or even shake everywhere. You might have a pit in your stomach or an emotion of fear about what will occur straight away.

On the off chance that you're confronted with danger, your body will get ready for one or the other battle or escape. At the point when we are worried, it's normal as far as we're concerned to feel nervous and experience difficulty focusing or thinking obviously. You could have considerations like "I will swoon," or "Get me out of here! I need to run!"

Dread is perhaps one of the most fundamental and basic emotions we have as people. Dread is a personal reaction to a detectable danger of risk, torment, or damage. At the point when somebody feels an emotion of dread it is typically an endurance intuition to assist them with keeping away from a perilous circumstance or if nothing else knows about the possible risk around them.

Dread advises you to run! While dread is a reaction to a current danger, nervousness is an inclination that is many times set off by anxiety toward something terrible occurring from here on out. Uneasiness is in many cases experienced despite the fact that there is no genuine danger, just an apparent one. Uneasiness might mean now is the ideal time to recapture some emotion of command over your Emotions or circumstance. It might likewise mean you really want to relinquish things that are not in your control.

The Job Emotions Play

Close-to-home mindfulness is the capacity to recognize and figure out your sentiments and Emotions . Quite possibly the main determinant of the way you connect with yourself as well as other people is your degree of profound mindfulness. It influences all aspects of your life, from how you feel, the decisions and how you deal with your Emotions of anxiety.

Individuals who are sincerely mindful are better ready to pay attention to other people and figure out their sentiments (this is sympathizing). They're additionally more alright with closeness since they understand what it seems like to be open about their own sentiments.

Individuals who are more on top of understanding sentiments and Emotions likewise have a better mental self-view and are less inclined to be genuinely vexed when something turns out badly.

Having the option to recognize your are Emotionat some random time empowers you to come to conclusions about how best to continue. You can choose whether to make a move or sit idle, yet basically, you will have a superior comprehension of what your choices are.

Likewise, distinguishing your Emotions precisely assists you with figuring out the significance of the paltry.

You figure out how to pay attention to your gut Emotions and not disregard what's happening within you.

1.The Voice Of Bitterness

At the point when we feel miserable we might encounter greatness in the heart and chest, and become sad and bound to

Ace your emotions

want to pull out from individuals. Misery can cause us to feel dormant and we probably won't have the option to focus very well on something besides our agony.

At the point when individuals feel bitterness or sadness they frequently experience unmistakable inclinations of void or gloom; considerations, for example, "this aggravation won't ever disappear" or "I'm isolated"; the motivation to pull out, rest or cry; trouble concentrating, and additionally contemplations about needing to keep away from life.

Misery is an inclination that can be set off by numerous occasions, for example, the deficiency of somebody close, the cutback of employment, and, surprisingly, the separation of a relationship.

The sensation of pity frequently lets us know that something is absent in our lives or that some misfortune or dissatisfaction has happened. Pity flags a requirement for solace and backing. It could imply that we want to deal with ourselves and permit ourselves an opportunity to mend.

2. Try not to Pass judgement on Your Emotions

The most vital phase in understanding your sentiments and Emotions is to figure out how to acknowledge them without judgement. This can be troublesome on the grounds that a considerable lot of us have been helped, that it's not alright to feel specific Emotions , like resentment or misery.

Be that as it may, all Emotions are helpful and significant. Sobbing, for instance, is a characteristic approach to relinquishing repressed Emotions and delivering pressure. This as well as crying really delivers synapses (like oxytocin and endorphins) that will assist with pushing you back to additional positive Emotions .

Ace your emotions

Being sincerely mindful doesn't mean dwelling on your sentiments, examining them constantly, or in any event, following up on them, yet essentially recognizing, tolerating, and handling them as they emerge.

Sentiments that are not communicated or perceived can be exceptionally disastrous over extensive stretches of time. They can prompt pressure and uneasiness, as well as medical conditions including coronary illness, sleep deprivation, migraines and stomach-related messes. Unsettled sorrow can prompt what is known as muddled distress which is significantly more excruciating and hard to process than the first aggravation.

At the point when we keep down our Emotions , they become disassociated from us and beyond our control. By bringing them into awareness, we can recognize them and direct our conduct all the more actually.

Attempt to relinquish the decisions you have about your sentiments, and acknowledge them as only a piece of being human. Really at that time could you at any point start the most common way of figuring out how to oversee them in a solid manner?

What Every Inclination Feels Like and Everything that They are Attempting To Say to You

In certain circumstances, you could experience issues naming what you're feeling. This might occur on the off chance that you're Emotion Overpowered by a few unmistakable inclinations, like sorrow or bitterness.

This situation assists with focusing on how your body is responding and what considerations are going through your brain. By naming these responses, you can start to distinguish

Ace your emotions

the inclination that is causing them. It could assist with asking yourself:

What is my body telling me?

In the event that you're overpowered and don't have the foggiest idea how you feel, focus on the thing your body is doing: Are your shoulders tense? Is it true that you are grasping your jaw or clench hands without acknowledging it?

How can my psyche let me know I'm feeling? You might encounter considerations, for example, "I feel like something awful is going to occur" or "This present circumstance is just a little ridiculous" Focus on these contemplations and check whether they assist you with distinguishing how you're feeling.

Then, ask yourself, "What are my Emotions attempting to tell me?" Each emotion has a directive for you, in the event that you require some investment to realise what it is. At the point when you become mindful of an inclination or feeling, make a stride back and attempt to comprehend what it implies.

It is likewise conceivable to encounter more than one emotion on the double.

For instance, you could at the same time feel outraged and hurt, or responsible and shame. At the point when this occurs, attempt to independently manage each inclination. At the point when your sentiments are clear, simpler to utilize the fitting survival methods will diffuse their adverse consequences.

The Voice Of Shock

At the point when you're amazed your heart speeds up and you might feel totally alert, mixed up and bleary-eyed. You might encounter a shock of energy all through the body. You

Ace your emotions

could feel frozen completely still or overpowered. You could have considerations like "I don't know what to do," or "I don't have the foggiest idea how to respond."

Shock is an inclination that can be set off by surprising or startling occasions/cooperations. Emotionshocked is typically established in the sensation of being surprised.

It can likewise be established in the sensation of nonpartisan or positive things out of the blue happening, for example, getting a commendation or getting an advancement at work. Shock lets you know that now is the right time to dial back and cycle data since something unforeseen has occurred.

The Voice Of Bliss

Bliss is typically set off by good occasions or connections that encourage you. At the point when you are cheerful you might encounter a sensation of happiness and delight. In some cases, bliss can be set off by the littlest thing like a commendation or completing a task on time.

Bliss signals you into things that are vital to you, for example, having good associations with others, acquiring new abilities or capacities, and Emotionlike you have a place.

Joy: Many individuals make progress toward joy, as it is a charming inclination joined by an emotion of prosperity and fulfilment. Joy is in many cases communicated by grinning or talking in an energetic manner of speaking.

Bitterness: We all experience misery from time to time. Somebody could communicate bitterness by crying, being calm, and additionally pulling out from others.

Kinds of misery incorporate distress, sadness, and dissatisfaction.

Dread: Dread can increment pulse, cause hustling considerations, or trigger the survival reaction. It very well may be a response to genuine or seen dangers. Certain individuals partake in the adrenaline rush that goes with dread through watching frightening motion pictures, riding thrill rides, or skydiving.

Disdain: Repugnance can be set off by an actual encounter, like seeing or smelling spoiling food, blood, or unfortunate cleanliness. Moral repugnance might happen when somebody sees someone else accomplishing something they see as improper or offensive.

Outrage: Outrage can be communicated with looks like glaring, hollering, or a rough way of behaving. Outrage can rouse you to make changes in your day-to-day existence, however, you want to track down a solid outlet to communicate outrage so it doesn't really hurt yourself or others.

Shock: Shock can be wonderful or disagreeable. You could open your mouth or wheeze when you're surprised.Shock, similar to fear, can set off the survival reaction.

Emotions , Sentiments, and Temperaments

In regular language, individuals frequently utilize the terms Emotions , sentiments, and temperaments reciprocally, yet these terms really mean various things. An inclination is regularly very fleeting, yet serious. Emotions are likewise liable to have an unmistakable and recognizable reason. For instance, subsequent to contradicting a companion over governmental issues, you could encounter outrage.

Emotions are responses to improvements, yet sentiments are what we experience because of Emotions . Sentiments are impacted by our impression of the circumstance, which is the reason a similar inclination can set off various sentiments among individuals encountering it

Ace your emotions

The Voices Of Responsibility and ShameGuilt

is an inclination about a singular activity one has committed. At the point when you feel remorseful it seems like a sharp agony in your heart, and you might end up needing to offer to set things straight with the individual you hurt. Culpability is a consequence of accomplishing something that disregards your very own ethical code or rules. At the point when individuals feel culpability, they frequently have considerations, for example, "I accomplished something awful," or "I ought to have accomplished something in an unexpected way."

Disgrace, then again, can feel like a significant burden overwhelming your shoulders, and you might want to stow away from others. Disgrace is a pessimistic inclination that spotlights oneself. "Oneself" is the kind of person you are personally. We feel disgraceful when we imagine that our identity as an individual is imperfect and damaged. At the point when individuals feel disgraced, they have considerations, for example, "I'm awful," or "I'm useless."

Disgrace can destructively affect your confidence and the emotions of your personality. The point when disgrace goes unattended in our life, it frequently causes us to feel unreliable, disliked and desolate. Driving away loved ones could somehow or another be strong.

Responsibility, then again, signals that what we did may have been off-base, however, our identity as an individual is dead on. It can assist us with the understanding that our way of behaving has harmed somebody or broken a significant relationship and may give the force want to apologize and accommodate

Record Your Contemplations and Emotions

Ace your emotions

You can work on tuning in and understanding sentiments and Emotions that you experience by getting into the propensity for recording your Emotions consistently, every time you feel something new or unique. This will assist you with recognizing your examples and give you knowledge of how you are Emotions After some time.

Self look at

What is causing me to feel as such?

In the event that you're Emotionrestless, what is causing it? Is there a troublesome undertaking approaching in your future that could prompt execution uneasiness? Assuming you're Emotionmiserable, for what reason would you say you are Emotions such? Is it true that you are watching a film or show that is inspiring emotion in you? What happened recently that could have caused the inclination?

Investigate what is going on and recognize what's setting off those sentiments. When you can perceive your triggers, you'll be more ready to stay away from future pessimistic sentiments, or if nothing else figure out how to actually adapt to them more.

Pessimistic considerations can likewise assume a significant part in moulding Emotions , and by and large, they really make the sentiments we experience because of them.

For instance: Assuming you think "I can't," or "I'll always be unable to do this," you could wind up feeling Restless, overpowered, and worried. Nonetheless, when you supplant those considerations with something like, "This is truly difficult, however, I'm ready to do my absolute best with it," you could wind up Emotions More sure and in charge.

To get familiar with the pessimistic reasoning that could be influencing your Emotions

Ace your emotions

•Talk about Your Thoughts

The most widely recognized way many individuals discharge gloomy sentiments is by discussing them or offering them to somebody they trust. You don't need to meticulously describe the situation, simply voicing without holding back the considerations that are upsetting you will assist with dispersing a portion of their force and make it more straightforward to acquire a more extensive point of view.

Talking and understanding sentiments and Emotions is likewise one of the most amazing ways of figuring them out. Frequently, when we are furious or apprehensive, the issue appears to be greater than it truly is. By talking things over with somebody who tunes in without making a decision about us or becoming protective, we can acquire knowledge of how to really determine what is going on.

•Grow Your Close home Jargon

Words matter. On the off chance that you're encountering areas of strength, pause for a minute to consider what to call it. In any case, don't stop there: Whenever you've recognized it, attempt to concoct two additional words that depict how you are feeling. You may be shocked to find a more profound inclination covered underneath the more clear one. It's similarly critical to do this with "positive" Emotions as well as "pessimistic" ones.

Fostering a bigger jargon for understanding sentiments and emotions can be useful. Making a rundown of Emotion Words and taking care of them from least upsetting to most troubling can assist you with distinguishing your inclination and subsequently what you really want.

Ace your emotions

Assuming you are Emotionirate, you could inquire as to whether you are "somewhat irritated," "aggravated", "incensed" or even "maddened." The word that you pick can assist you with distinguishing your beginning stage and the power of your inclination.

Then you can design as needs be and move toward settling or dealing with your sentiments. The right words illustrate what you're going through and assist you with better communicating those sentiments to other people.

See a specialist

In the event that you feel like not understanding sentiments and Emotions is beginning to obstruct exercises, for example, work, or everyday life, it very well might be an ideal opportunity to converse with somebody who is prepared to assist you with managing your sentiments in a methodical manner.

Advisors can assist you with grasping how explicit considerations, actual sensations, ways of behaving, and previous encounters cooperate to make sensations of nervousness, disgrace, and so on. They can likewise show you methodologies for "establishing" yourself when you begin to feel overpowered.

That finishes us off of this post on figuring out sentiments and Emotions .

Managing Emotions is a key initiative expertise. Also, naming our Emotions — what therapists call "marking" — is a significant initial phase in managing them really. Yet, it's harder than it sounds; a large number of us battle to recognize what precisely we are feeling, and frequently the clearest name isn't really the most reliable.

Ace your emotions

Outrage and stress are two of the Emotions we see most in the working environment — or if nothing else those are the terms we use for them most often. However, they are in many cases veils for more profound sentiments that we would be able and ought to portray in more nuanced and exact ways.

It's been shown that when individuals don't recognize and address their Emotions , they show lower prosperity and more actual side effects of pressure. On the other side, having the right jargon permits us to see the main problem in question — to take a muddled encounter, comprehend it all the more plainly and fabricate a guide to resolve the issue.

•think about the force of the inclination

We're well-suited to jump to essential descriptors like "furious" or "focused" in any event when our sentiments are undeniably less limited. It is important in your own self-appraisal whether you are irate or simply cantankerous, melancholy or recently frightened, happy or recently satisfied. As you mark your Emotions , likewise rate them on a size of 1 to 10 to check how profoundly or direly you are emotional.

• Work it out

Pennebaker's tests uncovered that individuals who expound on sincerely charged episodes experience an obvious expansion in their physical and mental prosperity. Besides, in an investigation of late laid-off labourers, he found that the people who dove into their sensations of embarrassment, outrage, uneasiness and relationship challenges were multiple times bound to have been re-utilized than those in control gatherings. The method involved with composing permitted them to acquire another viewpoint on their Emotions and to obviously grasp them and their suggestions more.

Ace your emotions

You can likewise utilise these three methodologies — expanding your jargon, noticing the power of an inclination and working it out — while attempting to more readily figure out someone else's Emotions . By really understanding what they are emotionally more exactly, you will be better prepared to answer in a helpful manner.

When you comprehend what you are feeling, then, at that point, you can all the more likely location and gain from those all the more precisely portrayed Emotions .

What makes somebody sincerely ignorant?

On the off chance that you feel withdrawn from your Emotions , there are a few reasons this may be the situation.

The connection hypothesis proposes how intently you clung to your essential guardians in adolescence can direct your profound accessibility as a grown-up.

"Genuinely far off, inaccessible, and dismissing connection figures over the course of growing up is many times a typical encounter for individuals who find recognizing and examining their Emotions testing," says Gabrielle Montana, an authorized proficient guide in Fitchburg, Wisconsin.

Assuming your guardians were sincerely detached or keeping, it's regular you could figure out how to demonstrate that in adulthood.

Injury

Roma Williams, an authorized marriage and family specialist in Houston, shows injury can forestall profound mindfulness by making somebody shut down inwardly.

This self-defensive state can keep you from emotional Emotions or remembering them in others.

Emotional well-being conditions

"There are sure psychological well-being conditions that can make somebody be genuinely ignorant," says Williams. "For instance, individuals with the marginal behavioural condition might experience issues controlling their Emotions and understanding what they are feeling."

Other psychological wellness conditions that could prevent you from understanding Emotions include:

Why is understanding Emotions significant?

Emotions might have a premise in endurance-situated learning, yet they likewise act as a significant device for building associations with others.

The expression "connect with" demonstrates you can relate to another person. Maybe you perceive what they're Emotion Since you've remembered in yourself.

Understanding Emotions can assist you with turning out to be more compassionate and can assist you with laying out an emotional trust.

Expertise can likewise help your own psychological prosperity.

That's what Montana alerts "When we can't recognize, adjust to, or draw in with our own Emotions , this can prompt:

unfortunate confidence

negative contemplations about self

searching for outlets to discover the help of some kind or another

Ace your emotions

"This eventually prompts pessimistic input circles and keeps us Emotion stuck."

Tips to distinguish and grasp your Emotions

There are various ways you can make progress toward figuring out Emotions .

Body checking

While you're Emotional inclination, connecting it to a body sensation can assist you with grasping it.

"Start with seeing the sensation in your body while watching a film or hearing a tune that you know causes bitterness, happiness or upset," recommends Celeste Labadie, an authorised marriage and family specialist in Stone, Colorado.

Whenever you've distinguished the sensations, you can ask yourself everything they're attempting to say to you

Then tune in for something extremely easy to emerge," says Labadie. "One more method for moving toward this is, 'On the off chance that I was a canine, what might thunder in my gut be telling me?' This will truly work on it and get you out of your coherent reasoning cerebrum."

Montana suggests utilizing a profound wheel, made without help from anyone else or tracked down on the web, that rundowns various Emotions and their going with sensations.

"It may not be that you don't have close-to-home mindfulness, but rather that all things considered, you don't approach the language you want to depict your profound experience," she says.

Close to home and Mental Compassion

Scientists recognize two kinds of compassion. Particularly in friendly brain research, compassion can be arranged as a profound or mental reaction. Close-to-home compassion comprises three separate parts, Hodges and Myers say. "The

Ace your emotions

first is Emotional similar Emotions to someone else … The subsequent part, individual pain, alludes to one's own sensations of trouble in light of seeing another's situation … The third close-to-home part, Emotion Sympathy for someone else, is the one most often connected with the investigation of compassion in brain research," they make sense of.

It is essential to take note that sensations of trouble related to profound compassion don't be guaranteed to reflect the Emotions of the other individual. That's what Hodges and Myers note, while compassionate individuals feel trouble when somebody falls, they aren't in a similar actual torment. This kind of sympathy is particularly important with regard to conversations of sympathetic human behaviour. There is a good relationship between Emotion Empathic concern and being willing to help other people. "A significant number of the most respectable instances of human way of behaving, including helping outsiders and demonised individuals, are remembered to have empathy roots,"

The subsequent part, individual pain, alludes to one's own sensations of misery because of seeing another's predicament … The third profound part, Emotion Sympathy for someone else, is the one most often connected with the investigation of compassion in brain science," they make sense of.

It is critical to take note that sensations of pain related with close to home sympathy don't be guaranteed to reflect the Emotions of the other individual. That's what Hodges and Myers note, while compassionate individuals feel trouble when somebody falls, they aren't in a similar actual torment. This kind of sympathy is particularly significant with regard to conversations of sympathetic human behaviour. There is a good relationship between Emotion Empathic concern and

Ace your emotions

being willing to help other people. "Large numbers of the most honourable instances of human way of behaving, including helping outsiders and slandered individuals, are remembered to have empathic roots," as indicated by Hodges and Myers. Banter remains concerned whether the motivation to help is situated in charitableness or personal circumstance.

The second kind of compassion is mental sympathy. This alludes to how well an individual can see and comprehend the Emotions of another. Mental compassion, otherwise called empathic exactness, includes "having more complete and precise information about the items in someone else's psyche, including the way that the individual feels," Hodges and Myers say. Mental compassion is more similar to expertise: People figure out how to perceive and comprehend others' close-to-home state as a method for handling Emotions and conduct. While it's not satisfactory precisely the way that people experience compassion, there is a developing collection of exploration on the subject.

How Would We Sympathise?

Specialists in the field of social neuroscience have created two speculations trying to acquire a superior comprehension of compassion. The first, Reproduction Hypothesis, "recommends that sympathy is conceivable in light of the fact that when we see someone else encountering an inclination, we 'mimic' or address that equivalent emotional ourselves so we can know firsthand what it seems like," as per Brain research Today.

There is an organic part to this hypothesis too. Researchers have found fundamental proof of "reflect neurons' ' that fire when people notice and experience feeling. There are too "portions of the mind in the average prefrontal cortex (liable for more significant level sorts of felt) that show crossover of actuation for both self-engaged and other-centred considerations and decisions," a similar article makes sense of.

A few specialists accept the other logical clarification of compassion in the finished resistance to the Reproduction Hypothesis. It's the Hypothesis of the Brain, the capacity to "comprehend what someone else is thinking and emotional view of rules for how one ought to think or feel," Brain research Today says. This hypothesis proposes that people can utilise mental manners of thinking to make sense of the psychological condition of others. By creating speculations about the human way of behaving, people can foresee or make sense of others' activities, as per this hypothesis.

While there is no unmistakable agreement, almost certainly, sympathy includes different cycles that integrate both programmed, profound reactions and learned calculated thinking. Contingent upon setting and circumstance,

Knowing the Egotist

Curiously, they likewise evaluated themselves as having more elevated levels of negative parts of self-centeredness, for example, being power-situated, incautious, pompous, and inclined to overstate their capacities. As such, egomaniacs know that they are narcissists. Analysing their information, they found that they could dependably distinguish egotists, basically utilising the inquiry: "How much do you concur with this assertion: 'I'm a narcissist. When the egomaniac realises you have sorted him out and when they have zero control over you, one of the normal egomaniac responses is to play on your close-to-home side. They will utilise every one of their contrivances to go after you, causing you to feel for them.

Ace your emotions

People with self-absorption tend not to like seeing others blissful. Everything you can manage is to remain firm on your limits, centre around the present and what satisfies you, and try not to get into contentions. They could attempt to hurt you to upset your tranquillity and legitimise their activities.

Individuals with selfishness tend not to like seeing others blissful. Everything you can manage is to remain firm on your limits, centre around the present and what fulfils you, and try not to get into contentions. They could attempt to hurt you to disturb your tranquillity and legitimise their actions. Type As can likewise be hazardous to egotists

In spite of the fact that they can be designated, type A group can likewise turn into an egotist's most dreaded fear. One of the main protections against dull characters is areas of strength for having yourself, and the type A group are generally mindful that they reserve the option to construct them.

Keep Up The Picture. ...

Earnestly Praise Them. ...

Go "No Contact" ...

Feed Their Self-image. ...

Keep The Trepidation alive. ...

Concur With Them. ...

Try not to Yield. ...

Keep quiet And Patient.

Contrasts in Character

Ace your emotions

Section 3

Empath, and Egotist

Empaths are something contrary to egotists. While individuals with the self-centred behavioural condition have no compassion and blossom with the requirement for reverence, empaths are exceptionally delicate and on top of others' Emotions . Empaths are "close-to-home wipes," who can retain sentiments from others very easily. Both an empath and egotist are extremely delicate people however in various ways. Empaths might incorporate what others are going through, faulting themselves for being not able to cheer others up. Furthermore, then again, egomaniacs will generally seriously despise analysis or sensations of inadequacy. The egotist can keep the empath in a pattern of profound or actual maltreatment and keep on crippling the empath and using them as the substitute for their own broken sentiments. Empaths will quite often incorporate sentiments and acknowledge blame. An empath frequently struggles with abandoning somebody and needs to accept that their sympathy will recuperate the self-involved person. Frequently when an empath faces an egomaniac with their terrible way of behaving, they can be met with fury and allegations that the empath isn't perceiving all the work they are placing in.

Sympathy versus Affectedness

Empaths feel for individuals, figure out their battles, and need to show up for them. Egotists, conversely, frequently respect themselves and have an emotion of self-importance, accepting that they are superior to every other person. They frequently go about as though they merit adoration and regard without giving it out.

1. Boundaries and Regard

Empaths frequently experience issues defining limits with others and may assume the weights of people around them. They understand a lot that they don't even for one second consider safeguarding themselves. In any event, not until it's past the point of no return.

Egomaniacs, then again, have no issues defining limits. These are not individuals you at any point need to stress over losing an excessive number of inquiries about "what's truly happening" or "why have you been so miserable recently?".

Indeed, they regard your limits since they simply couldn't care less.

2. Communication Style

You essentially will not need to consider how an empath is Emotion About something. They might be quieter in discussions and are in many cases able to comprehend where the speaker is coming from regarding experience.

Imparting empathically with an empath can very compensate, as they truly carve out the opportunity to tune in. As well as paying attention to you, don't be shocked on the off chance that they ask follow-up inquiries to all the more likely to identify.

Egomaniacs frequently talk in an exceptionally pretentious style, gloating about their achievements and patronising people around them. They are exceptionally conceited and will successfully be the focal point of consideration.

Since they are so egotistical, don't expect a discussion except if they can figure out how to make it about them. For instance,

Ace your emotions

you might attempt to enlighten them concerning your day, however, they will hinder you once they find a way to segway into something connected with them.

You might say," My little girl made her most memorable strides today!". Rather than saying congrats, the egomaniac companion might answer with, "So what, my kid emerged from my belly previously strolling. At point when I was two months old, I was at that point doing reverse flips in my lodging."

3. Need for Consideration

Both empaths and egotists need consideration, however, empaths need to give it out however much they get it.

They are continuously searching for ways of holding with and interfacing with individuals. They understand it gives them pleasure to have the option to help other people rest easier by thinking about themselves.

Egomaniacs likewise need consideration, yet they need to be the ones getting it. Each discussion is a way for them to discuss themselves, and they frequently couldn't care less about how the other individual is feeling.

They will take the necessary steps to stand out; regardless of whether that implies lying, controlling the circumstance, stirring something up, or with regards to specific world "pioneers", they might go similar to beginning a conflict on an honest nation or continually take steps to utilise atomic rockets.

4.. Taking care of Analysis

Empaths are for the most part very open to analysis and will attempt to gain from it. Keep in mind, these are individuals that are continuously endeavouring to associate with others. In this way, assuming somebody offers something that they see

Ace your emotions

as hard to hear, empaths will attempt to comprehend the reason why the individual said it and how they can gain from it. The last thing they believe should do is made somebody feel awful or make them struggle.

Egotists, then again, can't deal with analysis by any means. They frequently carry on in an unfriendly way and will frequently go on edge. They frequently become exceptionally upset and will answer with unfriendly words or even undermine actual viciousness. It is essential to recollect that egotists are unbelievably delicate and any analysis can be taken by and by.

5. Mindfulness

Empaths are extremely mindful, particularly with regard to their Emotions . They are continually assessing the way in which they are Emotions and where those sentiments are coming from. You might see empaths purchasing all the self-improvement guides at Barnes and Respectable or citing their number one holistic mentors or advisors.

Their #1 link channel is presumably OWN, where they can watch shows like Super Soul Sunday and Oprah's Lord Class. Empaths are continuously searching for ways of bettering themselves by diving deeper into their general surroundings.

Egomaniacs, then again, have almost no mindfulness. They frequently believe that they are wonderful simply how they are and won't actually engage in changing something important to them.

Regardless of whether somebody calls attention to a blemish in their character, egotists will just dismiss it as not being a joking matter. Their number one film is presumably The Wolf of Money Road or The Incomparable Gatsby, where they can see individuals very much like them pulling off absolutely everything.

Suppose you told an egomaniac their nose is running. They might fault you for giving them a cold, or blame you for being negative.

6. Real Thoughtfulness

Empaths are the absolute most considerate individuals you will at any point meet. They frequently make a special effort to help other people, regardless of whether it implies burdening themselves. These are the sort of individuals that will purchase occasion presents or arbitrary ones at different seasons without anticipating one consequently. Basically, they simply need to cause others to feel better and feel that bliss back consequently.

Egotists, then again, are not fit for authentic thoughtfulness. Certainly, they might accomplish something pleasant for you now and again, yet it is ordinarily in view of a plan. They are searching for something consequently or a method for getting something from you. They might get you supper, yet ensure that you realise it was them who paid for itself and anticipate an acknowledgement consequently of some sort.

They might begin being pleasant to you once they understand you just got a major advancement or have a renowned companion. Without a doubt, they might offer their assistance or back to you in a period of scarcity, yet it is many times more about how it makes them look as opposed to genuinely needing to show up for you.

7.Love and Connections

For empaths, love looks like being sacrificial and putting the necessities of their accomplice before their own. They are faithful and consistently endeavour to construct areas of

Ace your emotions

strength for the individual they care about. Empaths frequently end up needing to associate on a profound level with the goal that they can ensure their accomplice is genuinely perceived.

Egomaniacs, be that as it may, have an entirely unexpected perspective on adoration. They need somebody that will continually make them feel better and do right by them. They are searching for somebody to venerate them and be there to serve their requirements, not the reverse way around.

Egomaniacs will generally bounce from one relationship to another looking for the ideal individual that can thoroughly take care of them without objection. Try not to be shocked in the event that an egomaniac talks truly about "exchanging" their companion once they go downhill, put on weight, or lose their looks

8. Mental and Profound Wellbeing

Empaths are extraordinarily in line with their psychological and close-to-home well-being. They frequently comprehend how things like injury, undesirable past connections, or even youth encounters have formed the manner in which they think and feel today. They can frequently ponder explicit occasions that made them excessively worried about other people.

Try not to be shocked assuming they start a soup kitchen and concede that they were once in a comparable situation to those they are making a difference.

Empaths will carve out an opportunity to recuperate and figure out through these problems to better themselves and their associations with others.

Egotists, then again, frequently couldn't care less about tending to any psychological or profound medical problems they might have. They just forget about them as being insignificant or something that can be managed later.

Keep in mind, they consider themselves to be great - it's every other person with the issue! On the off chance that they run over a gathering in a group, they will fault individuals for impeding their vehicle.

They are not ready to investigate the base of any issues, and frequently disregard or rationalise all things being equal.

9. Hard working attitude

Empaths flourish in any work that permits them to help other people. They are much of the time self-starters who endeavour to ensure they take care of business properly and needn't bother with a great deal of inspiration or acknowledgement from others. They are additionally imaginative issue solvers who like to break new ground and think of arrangements that genuinely benefit all interested parties.

Egomaniacs, then again, will just do what's to their greatest advantage and will frequently pursue faster routes to get what they need. Obviously, that doesn't mean egotists don't succeed!

Going against the norm, they can frequently find success in their vocations, particularly in the corporate world, which is much of the time relentless. In any case, it is generally on the grounds that they will take the necessary steps - regardless of whether it implies offending others - to excel.

Ace your emotions

Empath Versus Egotist Character

If empaths and egomaniacs were two of a kind, empaths would be the side that is looking up. They are magnanimous, mindful, and continuously able to loan some assistance to those out of luck - regardless of whether it implies troubling themselves.

Egotists are many times on the other side, searching for somebody to lift their confidence and do right by them.

Anyway, are the wheels in your mind turning as you keep thinking about whether you fit one of these character qualities? There are different tests accessible that can give you knowledge of your character type and assist with directing you in understanding yourself better.

You can step through the examination for self-centeredness and the one for empaths in only a couple of moments on the web. On occasion, you might have shown the two characteristics recorded above - everyone makes mistakes and sympathetic versus egomaniac characters are no special case.

The key is to perceive when you are inclining more toward one side and to do whatever it takes to ensure both your empath and self-involved sides stay adjusted with the goal that you can be your best self.

With the right comprehension of these two character attributes, we can all encourage more merciful and sympathetic associations with ourselves and the people around us

Dealing with Your Emotions

God Provided You Emotions on Motivation! Our Emotions assume a fundamental part in living cheerful, solid, fruitful lives. All Emotions , from adoration and delight to outrage and dread, have a significant part to play in grasping ourselves as well as other people. They assist us with finding the miracles of this life as well as caution us when we are in harm's way. Gloomy Emotions like trepidation, trouble, and outrage are an essential piece of life and here and there we battle with how to really manage them. It very well may be enticing to follow up on the thing you're Emotionimmediately, however that frequently doesn't fix what is happening that caused the Emotions . As a matter of fact, it might prompt more issues to manage not too far off.

A portion of the destructive ways that individuals manage pessimistic Emotions :

Forswearing

Forswearing is the point at which an individual will not acknowledge that anything is off-base or that help might be required. At the point when individuals reject that they are having tricky sentiments, those sentiments can restrain to a point that an individual winds up "detonating" or carrying on in a hurtful way.

Withdrawal

Withdrawal is the point at which an individual would rather not be near, or partake in exercises with others. This is not the

Ace your emotions

same as needing to be separated from everyone else occasionally and can be an admonition indication of misery. Certain individuals might pull out in light of the fact that being around others takes an excessive amount of energy, or they feel overpowered. Others might pull out on the grounds that they don't think others like them or believe they should be near. Now and again, individuals who have ways of behaving that they are embarrassed about may pull out so others don't learn about the thing they are doing. Yet, withdrawal brings its own concerns: outrageous forlornness, misjudging, outrage, and twisted thinking. We really want to communicate with others to keep us adjusted.

Harassing

Harassing is the point at which an individual proposes power, danger, or derision to show control over others. Individuals regularly partake in harassing conduct since they don't feel better about themselves and causing another person to feel terrible helps them have an improved outlook on themselves or feel less alone. It is unsafe for both the domineering jerk and the individual being harassed and doesn't resolve basic issues.

Self-Mischief

Self-mischief can take many structures including: cutting, starving oneself, pigging out then vomiting, or partaking in a hazardous way of behaving. Many individuals are self-hurt since they feel like it gives them command over profound agony. While self-hurting might bring impermanent alleviation, these ways of behaving can become habit-forming and can lead individuals to be wilder and in more prominent agony than at any time in recent memory.

Substance Use

Ace your emotions

Substance use is the utilisation of liquor and different medications to cause an individual to feel far improved or numb about excruciating circumstances. Liquor and medication use can harm the mind, making it need higher measures of substances to get a similar impact. This can exacerbate troublesome sentiments and at times, prompt self-destructive considerations or dependence. On the off chance that you are worried about your own or another person's utilisation of medications or liquor, converse with a capable grown-up immediately to find support.

Stage 1: Delay.

This step is significant in light of the fact that as opposed to following up on sentiments immediately, you stop yourself and thoroughly consider things. Build up to 100 or say the letter set in reverse.

Stage 2: Recognize What You're Feeling.

For instance, would you say you are distraught at somebody, or would you say you are miserable in light of the fact that your sentiments were wounded by what they did? Whatever you are feeling, having that impression is alright.

Stage 3: Think.

Since you have taken a couple of seconds to sort out what precisely it is that you are feeling, contemplate how you can affect yourself better.

Stage 4: Help.

Make a move to help yourself in view of what you concocted in the "Think" step.

Tips

Peruse the narrative of somebody you respect

Watch an interesting YouTube video

Play with a creature

Watch a film you cherished when you were more youthful

Revamp your room

Make a rundown of spots you need to travel

Address Your Fundamental Requirements

Eat a solid bite.

Drink a glass of water.

Wash up.

Sleep.

Process Sentiments

Draw how you're feeling.

Make an appreciation list

Punch a pad.

Shout.

Allow yourself to cry.

Tear the paper into little pieces.

•**Vent**. Venting isn't equivalent to requesting help, it's making a move to discuss your thoughts without holding back. We do this normally when we talk with somebody we can believe about whatever is disturbing us. You can also vent by constructing a write up to the person l who piss you off. Keep the letter for two or three days and afterwards destroy it. Stick to pen and paper — utilising virtual entertainment when you are exceptionally close to home can be enticing, however, you could say something you lament.

•**Critical thinking**

Make a rundown of answers for issues - it can assist with conceptualising with a companion of a relative.

Ace your emotions

Make a rundown of your assets. There are a lot of things about you that are marvellous, regardless of how down you are.

•Chipping in/Thoughtful gestures

Accomplish something decent for somebody you know.

•Help an outsider.

•Volunteer your time.

•Side interests/Stress Relievers

•Discover some new information - there are instructional exercises for a wide range of side interests on the web.

•Make - attempt an art project, variety, paint, or draw. Welcome a companion to go along with you for added fun.

•Compose - you could compose a story, a sonnet, or a passage in a diary.

•Get dynamic - moving, running, or playing a game are decent ways of getting rolling.

•Play a computer game.

•Get a plant and begin a nursery.

•Unwinding Activities

•Practice gut breathing - put one hand on your stomach and begin to gradually breathe in. As you take in, envision an inflatable in your stomach topping off and keep on breathing in until the inflatable is extremely full. Put your other hand on your heart, feel your pulse, and pause your breathing for 5 seconds. Presently let your breath out leisurely for 10 seconds - feel your gut straighten like an emptying inflatable. Rehash this cycle 4 or multiple times and you ought to see your heartbeat delayed down and your muscles unwind.

Attempt moderate muscle unwinding - grasp your toes for a count of 5, then, at that point, loosen up them for a count of 5, then, at that point, move to your calves, then your thighs, then,

Ace your emotions

at that point, your abs, then, at that point, your arms, then, at that point, your neck.

•Play with Play-Doh.

•Take a walk - feel the ground under your feet and the air on your skin. Centre around your faculties.

Track down a directed reflection on YouTube.

•Do yoga - you can find recordings on request utilising your television or on the web.

•Peruse a book.

•Pay attention to music, a web recording, or a book recording.

•Turn off - switch off your telephone, tablet, or potentially PC for an hour or thereabouts.

•Request Help

•Text a companion.

•Ask somebody to simply sit with you.

•Call a relative.

•Converse with a grown-up you trust

Opening the Force of The ability to understand individuals on a deeper level

Perceiving, evaluating and communicating Emotions really is a fundamental ability for making sound connections and making progress in both expert and individual life. Being sincerely savvy assists with better grasping ourselves as well as other people, making a more adjusted and satisfied life. By understanding Emotions , it's feasible to foster better relational abilities, increment mindfulness and oversee pressure in better ways. Additionally, recognizing and understanding the Emotions of others can assist with making more grounded connections and exploring testing circumstances all the more successfully. Great profound administration includes figuring out how to control Emotions ,

Ace your emotions

express them suitably and differentially resolve clashes. With these abilities, it tends to be feasible to make more significant associations and accomplish more prominent fulfilment in both expert and individual lives.

Register today to recognize, comprehend and successfully deal with Emotions to assemble strong connections and prevail at work and throughout everyday life.

The capacity to understand people on a deeper level is a captivating and progressively significant point in this day and age. Have you at any point felt overpowered by your Emotions or attempted to comprehend and interface with others on a more profound level? Provided that this is true, you're in good company. Many individuals end up battling with the capacity to understand people on a deeper level, yet fortunately, expertise can be created and sharpened after some time.

At its centre, the ability to appreciate people on a profound level is tied in with having the option to perceive, comprehend, and deal with your own Emotions , as well as those of others. It's the capacity to involve Emotions to direct your considerations and activities in a good manner and to fabricate solid, significant associations with people around you.

Studies have shown that capacity to understand people on a profound level is a critical indicator of outcomes in both individual and expert settings. Individuals with a high ability to appreciate anyone on a deeper level are better ready to oversee pressure, impart successfully, and work cooperatively with others. They're likewise bound to be versatile even with difficulties and to return from misfortunes.

Ace your emotions

Creating the ability to understand individuals at their core is a continuous cycle, and one requires practice, tolerance, and industriousness. Yet, with the right outlook and devices, anybody can figure out how to develop these abilities and receive the many rewards that accompany the capacity to understand individuals on a profound level.

So whether you're hoping to work on your own connections, upgrade your vocation possibilities, or just increase a more profound comprehension of yourself and the people around you, the capacity to understand individuals at their core is a point certainly worth investigating. So how about we make a plunge and begin investigating the entrancing universe of the capacity to understand individuals on a deeper level together?

"Individuals will fail to remember what you said, individuals will fail to remember what you did, yet individuals will always remember how you affected them." - Maya Angelou

The Five Parts of The ability to understand individuals on a deeper level

What precisely does the ability to understand people at their core resemble and by?

The capacity to understand people on a deeper level is a complicated development that includes a scope of abilities and capacities connected with insight, handling, and the board of Emotions . While there are a few distinct models of the capacity to understand people on a profound level, one of the most generally acknowledged is the model proposed by Daniel Goleman, which distinguishes five vital parts of the capacity to appreciate individuals on a profound level. These

Ace your emotions

parts are mindfulness, self-guideline, inspiration, compassion, and interactive abilities.

1. Practice mindfulness

Mindfulness is the underpinning of the ability to appreciate people on a profound level. Creating mindfulness includes perceiving and figuring out one's own Emotions , assets, and shortcomings. One method for rehearsing mindfulness is to diary your Emotions and encounters. Take time every day to consider your contemplations and sentiments, and record them in a diary. This can assist you with perceiving designs in your Emotions and ways of behaving, and foster a more profound comprehension of yourself.

One more method for rehearsing mindfulness is to request criticism from others. Ask confided-in companions or partners for genuine criticism about your assets and shortcomings. This can assist you with distinguishing regions where you really want to improve and foster a more exact comprehension of how others see you.

2. Foster sympathy

Sympathy is the capacity to comprehend and connect with the Emotions and encounters of others. Creating compassion includes effectively paying attention to other people, perceiving and answering their Emotions , and taking into account their points of view. One method for creating compassion is to rehearse undivided attention. This includes completely zeroing in on the speaker, staying away from interruptions, and posing inquiries to explain their contemplations and sentiments. This can assist you with fostering a more profound comprehension of the speaker's viewpoint, and answer in a way that is humane and steady.

3. Search out new encounters

Ace your emotions

Searching out new encounters can be a strong method for creating the capacity to understand people at their core. Encountering new things can assist you with creating more noteworthy mindfulness, Constructing compassion, and fostering a more nuanced comprehension of your general surroundings. This can include attempting new side interests or exercises, going to new spots, or taking part in new friendly or expert encounters.

4. Practice appreciation

Appreciation is an integral asset for creating the capacity to understand people at their core. Rehearsing appreciation includes zeroing in on the positive parts of your life, and communicating appreciation for individuals and encounters that give you pleasure and satisfaction. Appreciation can assist with moving your viewpoint from one of need and pessimism to one of overflow and inspiration. By zeroing in on the beneficial things in your day-to-day existence, you can develop an emotion of satisfaction and bliss, even in troublesome times.

There are numerous ways of rehearsing appreciation, from keeping a day-to-day appreciation diary to just pausing for a minute every day to consider the things you are grateful for. You can likewise offer thanks to others through verbal or composed messages, or by performing thoughtful gestures and administration. By making appreciation a standard piece of your life, you can foster a more certain and sincerely keen mentality, and fabricate more grounded, additional satisfying associations with others

5. Construct solid connections

Building solid connections is a basic part of the capacity to understand individuals at their core. Creating solid connections includes being available and mindful, imparting reality, and fostering an emotion of trust and compatibility with others. One method for building solid connections is to rehearse undivided attention. This includes completely zeroing in on the speaker, keeping away from interruptions, and posing inquiries to explain their considerations and sentiments. This can assist you with fostering a more profound comprehension of the speaker's point of view, and answer in a way that is humane and strong.

One more method for building solid connections is to foster an emotion of trust and compatibility with others. This can include sharing individual stories or encounters, exhibiting dependability and consistency, and offering backing and consolation. Creating solid connections can assist you with building a strong organisation of companions and partners, and encourage an emotional feeling of having a place and association.

6. Practice close to the home guideline

The close-to-home guideline includes perceiving and dealing with one's own Emotions . Creating close-to-home guidelines includes perceiving when you are areas of strength for encountering, and creating methodologies to deal with those Emotions in a solid and helpful manner. One method for rehearsing close-to-home guidelines is to foster care practice. This includes zeroing in on the current second and noticing your considerations and Emotions without judgment. This can assist you with creating more prominent mindfulness and close-to-home guideline abilities

Section 5

Figuring out Emotions guidelines

Emotion Guideline concerns how individuals deal with close-to-home insight for individual and social purposes. It is a mind-boggling and complex interaction and is normatively significant in light of the fact that it is vital to social skill, mental prosperity, and hazard for full of Emotion Psychopathology. The improvement of the Emotion Guideline depends on early neurobiological development, formed by unstable distinction, and directed by the small kid's reasonable comprehension of feeling, methodologies of Emotion The executives, and oneself. It is additionally directed by friendly impacts: parental training, displaying, direct mediations, discussion, the nature of the parent-youngster relationship, and the novel impacts of companions and kin.

Emotion Guideline includes the change of profound reactions through the enrollment of methodologies that impact specific phases of the emotional process. such groups of Emotion Guideline methodologies, coordinated as far as the phase of the emotional process that they influence. Note that albeit the objective to control one's Emotions and the methodologies used to do so could hypothetically be initiated and work verifiably and consequently, practically all neuroscience investigations of Emotion Guideline have zeroed in on procedures that are unequivocally spurred, signalled, and executed.

The most groundbreaking groups of procedures, circumstance choice and change, involve endeavours to impact the sorts of circumstances that one will insight into or to alter important elements of those circumstances once you are in them. Then, consideration sending includes coordinating consideration toward or away from elements of a given circumstance, as while diverting oneself. From that point forward, mental change systems focus on our examinations, altering the manners in which we ponder a way to improve to change its close-to-home effect. The prototypical mental change system, reappraisal, includes intentionally transforming one's understanding of or potentially unique interaction to a boost. At long last, reaction adjustment methodologies target and regulate the conducting part of the close-to-home reaction, for instance, profound looks.

Concentrate on discoveries likewise have suggestions for programmed Emotion Guidelines.

To be sure, a third report gives proof that when given no particular guideline directions, guys and females really do utilise various procedures, and contrast in their mind enactment. During an undertaking where members were furnished with the overall guidance to downregulate their pessimistic profound reaction to close-to-home upgrades, Mak and colleagues65 found that for the guideline of gloomy inclination, guys showed more grounded enactment in the horizontal prefrontal cortex, front cingulate gyrus, and fleeting cortex. Conversely, females just had more grounded actuation in the average prefrontal cortex contrasted with guys. The creators recommend that the cerebrum locales selected by females to control pessimistic inclination were more connected with emotion handling, while those areas enlisted by guys were more connected with mental handling. This was in accordance with self-report appraisals posts can,

Ace your emotions

by which females revealed utilising more Emotion Centred survival methods while guys utilised more mental.

Notwithstanding distinctions in sexual orientation in effortful or mental Emotion Guideline, neuroimaging research gives some proof that there might be distinctions in sexual orientation in the more programmed and obvious Emotion Guideline processes that are locked in during openness to profound improvements. Without a doubt, various neuroimaging reads offer help for the idea that guys might participate in more productive programmed Emotion Administrative cycles than females. The examinations by Williams and associates and Thomas and colleagues, described above, propose that the component hidden expanded reactivity in females to fear upgrades could include supported limbic action, while guys answer in basically the same manner as females at first, however, recuperate all the more rapidly with limbic action lessening. That is, in guys, administrative components may be locked in more rapidly to hose emotional responses. Kempton and partners detailed diminished amygdala action in guys during the quiet marking of dread face boosts and proposed that this might reflect more prominent prefrontal restraint of amygdala movement related to programmed Emotion Guideline that is locked in during express inclination naming. Koch and partners utilised a functioning memory task during openness to unsavoury scents, by which task execution was remembered to cause programmed Emotion Administrative systems in members. The creators observed that the cooperation was related to more prominent male enactment in a front-parietal-cingulate network, though females showed more enactment in the orbitofrontal cortex and amygdala. In guys, the cooperation was related to locales regularly embroiled in fruitful Emotion Guideline, proposing that guys could participate in more compelling mental profound joining and subsequently Emotion Guideline. For sure, other work by these creators recommends that initiation of the fronto-parietal-cingulate network is related to a more viable programmed Emotion Guideline.

Emotion Guideline comprises the inner and outer cycles engaged with observing, assessing, and changing profound responses (particularly their force and fleeting highlights, like the speed of beginning and recuperation) to achieve one's objectives. Emotion Guideline is a significant point in the field of socioemotional improvement as a result of its hypothetical and functional ramifications .Hypothetically,Emotion Administrative cycles consolidate individual objectives, parental socialisation processes, cultural qualities, and social convictions into the development of profound life, and add to how individuals are genuinely particular yet additionally share close-to-home characteristics in various gatherings. For all intents and purposes, research on the advancement of the Emotion Guideline is critical to planning intercessions that can assist youngsters and grown-ups with issues related to Emotion dysregulation, including misery, uneasiness, hostility, and relationship unsettling influences. All the more, by and large, research on this subject tends to the difficulties of enrolling close-to-home responses valuably into versatile social working.

The meaning of the Emotion Guideline given above features that administrative cycles can be engaged with overseeing good as well as gloomy Emotions , (for example, smothering giggling while hearing a joke at a serious occasion), and can

Ace your emotions

include how others manage one's Emotions as well as one's own self-administrative endeavours. Emotion Guidelines by others are, obviously, particularly critical to babies and small kids. This meaning of Emotion Guideline additionally highlights that Emotion is overseen by changing its power and its transient elements (like its heightening, decline, or liability). People self-direct to diminish the power of sensations of misery, for instance, or to impede the quick heightening of outrage when incited, and it is the escalated and worldly highlights of emotion that are many times normal for Emotion-related psychopathology like melancholy.

Emotion Guidelines are significant for achieving one's objectives. This is reliable with the user perspective on Emotion Prior depicted and is significant for understanding how and why people deal with their Emotions as they do. In the formative examination, grown-ups may misperceive kids as sincerely dysregulated in circumstances where youngsters are working very well as profound strategists. Various objectives can direct Emotion Administrative endeavours, and different self-administrative methodologies can serve various objectives in various circumstances. A youngster who is being undermined by a friend, for instance, may deal with Emotions distinctively to achieve the prompt objective of deflecting the domineering jerk (e.g., crying noisily to inspire help) or to prevent future terrorising (e.g., controlling trepidation and improving resentment to shield oneself). The adequacy of elective Emotion Administrative procedures in achieving objectives depends, obviously, on the presence of others and the kid's associations with them, social qualities (e.g., Nepalese youngsters, are associated to stay away from any statement of gloomy Emotions), and numerous different variables.

In certain conditions of personal misfortune, the self-administrative test looked at by youngsters is that there are no ideal techniques for adapting to the close-to-home requests they face. Their Emotion Administrative procedures are logical, in this manner, to include innate compromises that buy quick adapting at the expense of long haul trouble, and which eventually may increment as opposed to reducing their close-to-home issues. A portion of the issues looked at by manhandled youngsters examined before, for instance, get from their touchiness to indications of grown-up outrage that empowers them to expect an oppressive experience to come, yet, in addition, renders them more inclined to be socially improper, forceful and direct with others. Similarly, youngsters with nervousness issues dedicate significant self-administrative work to keeping away from experiences with tension-inciting boosts, however, in doing so they acquire prompt close-to-home help at the expense of long-haul broken conduct. Seen in this light, the Emotion Guideline for kids in states of personal misfortune should be visible as a situation with two sides.

Formative changes in Emotion Guidelines give huge commitments to social and profound capability. Though a baby might cry wildly, the little child can look for help from others, the preschooler can ponder and discuss her sentiments, the young kid can divert consideration and utilise other intentional techniques to lessen trouble or nervousness, and the juvenile can bring out private methodologies (like paying attention to most loved music) that deal with the feeling. Numerous formative advances in the abilities of Emotion

Ace your emotions

Guideline represent these changes. With expanding age, kids come out as comfortable with and embrace socio cultural assumptions for profound articulations, particularly in open settings. They take care of dealing with their own good and gloomy sentiments. Their collection of self-started methodologies for dealing with Emotions develops, from an underlying dependence on conduct strategies that frequently depend on friendly help (e.g., looking for help; abstaining from sincerely stimulating occasions) to expanding utilisation of mentalistic techniques of Emotionself-guideline (e.g., attentional redirection; mental reappraisal). Over the long haul, besides, kids show expanding broadness, refinement, and adaptability in their utilisation of various Emotions Guideline techniques and are equipped for adjusting favoured procedures to the requests of the circumstance, subbing more successful methodologies after others have demonstrated insufficient, and in any event, utilising numerous systems when required. Kids additionally foster systems that are more powerful in dealing with specific Emotions (like apprehension) than others (like displeasure). The improvement of the Emotion Guideline is likewise founded on fostering comprehension of feeling, developing abilities to screen one's sentiments and evaluate the viability of self-administrative endeavours, and integrating the Emotionself-guideline into a more extensive assortment of conditions, (for example, upgrading critical thinking adequacy).

As noted before, the improvement of the Emotion Guideline is likewise connected with mental health, particularly with the sluggish development of the region of the prefrontal cortex that expects a huge impact on Emotion The executives. In any case, as prior noted, many mind frameworks are commonly compelling in Emotion Excitement and guideline, and that implies that cortical cerebrum locales pertinent to Emotionself-guideline are likewise affected by the action of cerebrum structures related to Emotion Actuation. For kids and grown-ups who experience the ill effects of Emotion Related psychopathology that includes changes in ordinary hormonal and neurobiological cycles related to feeling, the adequacy of prefrontal and other cortical regions associated with Emotionself-guideline is dulled due to the impacts on these areas of lower Emotion processes that have been impacted by psychopathology.

The investigation of the Emotion Guideline spices up the field of socioemotional improvement on account of the significant issues it raises concerning how close to-home experience is exclusively and socially developed, and due to its significant viable ramifications for understanding the starting points and treatment of Emotion-related psychopathology. As this short conversation has likewise delineated, the investigation of the Emotion Guideline is likewise interestingly integrative, including neurobiology, mental turn of events, social getting it, social qualities, individual objectives, and various other formative impacts.

Consequently, a modest bunch of neuroimaging concentrates on helping distinctions in sexual orientation in the brain relating to both oblivious (i.e., programmed) and cognizant (i.e., effortful) Emotion Guideline processes. Given the rising acknowledgement that deficiencies in the Emotion Guideline (especially expanded utilisation of maladaptive strategies61) are a trademark element of various psychological illnesses for which there are stamped distinctions in sexual orientation in commonness and presentation,69 further work on distinctions in sexual orientation in the brain hardware of various kinds of Emotion Guideline will be significant.

Emotions are a typical piece of daily existence. We feel disappointed when we're stranded in rush-hour gridlock. We feel miserable when we miss our friends and family. We can blow up when somebody lets us down or effectively harms us. While we hope to feel these Emotions routinely, certain individuals begin to encounter Emotions that are more unpredictable. They feel better upsides and worse low points, and these pinnacles and valleys start to influence their lives. People who experience extreme Emotions might end up quiet one second and afterwards miserable or furious the following. While many of us can have times when our Emotions go wild, for certain individuals it happens routinely. Their quickly changing Emotions can make them do and make statements they later lament. They might harm connections or hurt their believability with others.

There can be various reasons that somebody fails to keep a grip on their Emotions . They might be hereditarily inclined toward these fast changes. They might in all likelihood never have seen great close-to-home guidelines demonstrated or mastered the abilities. They might let go completely when they experience triggers for negative circumstances that occurred previously. There can likewise be actual changes that make an individual fail to keep a grip on their Emotions , for example, depletion or a drop in glucose.

Not a great explanation for the close-to-home instability, fortunately, we can learn better self-guideline. We can all profit from learning systems to get a handle on our Emotions .

Ace your emotions

A profound guideline is a capacity to all the more likely control our close-to-home state.

What are close-to-home control and guidelines?

Profound control and guideline are making any move that adjusts the power of a close-to-home insight. It doesn't mean smothering or keeping away from Emotions . With profound guideline abilities, you can impact which Emotions you have as well as how you express them.

At last, it alludes to the capacity to apply command over our Emotions through a great many methodologies successfully.

Certain individuals are greater at controlling their Emotions than others. They are high in ability to understand anyone on a deeper level and know about both their inside encounters and the sensations of others. While it might appear as though they're simply "normally quiet," these individuals experience gloomy sentiments as well. They've recently evolved survival techniques that permit them to self-manage troublesome Emotions.

Fortunately, profound self-guideline is certainly not a static characteristic. Emotion Guideline abilities can be acquired and worked on after some time. Figuring out how to oversee negative encounters can help your psychological and actual well-being.

For what reason are close-to-home guidelines significant?

As grown-ups, we are supposed to deal with our Emotions in manners that are socially OK and assist us with exploring our lives. At the point when our Emotions get the better of us, they can create issues.

Many elements can hinder close-to-home guidelines. These incorporate our convictions about gloomy Emotions or an absence of profound guideline abilities. In some cases,

Ace your emotions

unpleasant circumstances can bring out particularly strong Emotions .

One of the manners in which that profound unpredictability can hurt us incorporates the effect it can have on our associations with others. For instance, when we can't as expected to moderate our indignation, we are probably going to make statements that hurt people around us and influence them to pull away. We might lament the things we've said or need to invest energy in fixing connections.

As well as adversely affecting our connections, a powerlessness to get a grip on our Emotions can likewise hurt us. Emotions Overpowering bitterness can bring down prosperity and cause superfluous affliction. Living with complete trepidation can hinder our capacity to face challenges and have new valuable encounters.

5 Emotions Guideline abilities you ought to dominate

There are various abilities that can help us self-control our Emotions .

1. Make space

Emotions happen quickly. We don't think "presently I will be irate" — we are simply unexpectedly grip jawed and enraged. So the main expertise in controlling troublesome Emotions , the gift we can give ourselves, is to stop. Calmly inhale. Dial back the second among trigger and reactions.

2. Seeing what you feel

Similarly, significant expertise includes the capacity to become mindful of what you're feeling. Dr Judson Brewer, MD PhD suggests rehearses for turning out to be more inquisitive about your own actual responses. Check out yourself and consider: in which parts of your body would you

Ace your emotions

say you are seeing sensations? Is your stomach vexed? Is your heart hustling? Do you feel strain in your neck or head?

Your actual side effects can be signs of what you are encountering inwardly. Asking into what is befalling you genuinely can likewise divert your concentration and permit a portion of the power of the emotion to disappear.

3. Naming what you feel

In the wake of seeing what you feel, the capacity to name it can assist you with overseeing what's going on. Ask yourself: what might you call the Emotions you're feeling? Is it outrage, trouble, disillusionment, or hatred? What else is it? One number emotion that frequently stows away underneath others is dread.

A considerable lot of us feel more than each emotion in turn, so make sure to have numerous Emotions you may feel. In the event that you feel dread, what are you terrified of? On the off chance that you feel outraged, what are you irate about or toward? Having the option to name your Emotions will assist you to draw one stage nearer to imparting your Emotions to other people.

4. Tolerating the inclination

Emotions are an ordinary and regular piece of how we answer circumstances. As opposed to whipping yourself for being Emotionfurious or terrified, perceive that your profound responses are legitimate. Attempt to rehearse self-sympathy and give yourself effortlessness. Perceive that encountering Emotions is an ordinary human response.

5. Rehearsing care

Care helps us "live at the time" by focusing on what is inside us. Utilise your faculties to see what's going on around you in nonjudgmental ways. These abilities can assist you with

Ace your emotions

remaining cool-headed and try not to participate in pessimistic idea designs when you are amidst personal agony.

5. Rehearsing care

Care helps us "live at the time" by focusing on what is inside us. Utilise your faculties to see what's going on around you in nonjudgmental ways. These abilities can assist you with remaining cool-headed and try not to participate in pessimistic idea designs when you are amidst personal agony.

systems that can assist you with directing your Emotions

There are various Emotion Guideline techniques that individuals can dominate to construct their adapting abilities. It is vital to consider which methodologies are generally valuable and which ones to stay away from.

There are two general classifications of profound guidelines. The first is reappraisal: changing our opinion on something to change our reaction. The second is concealment, which is connected to additional adverse results. Research shows that disregarding our Emotions is related to disappointment and unfortunate prosperity.

We should take a gander at procedures that can assist with dealing with Emotions in a sound and supportive manner.

1. Recognize and diminish triggers

You shouldn't attempt to stay away from gloomy Emotions — or fear them. However, you likewise don't need to continue to place yourself in a circumstance that welcomes disagreeable Emotions Begin to search for examples or elements that are available when you begin to major areas of strength for feel. This requires some interest and trustworthiness. Accomplishing something cause you to feel little? Compelling Emotions frequently spring up out of our

Ace your emotions

firmly established uncertainties, particularly the ones we stow away. What's going on around you and what previous encounters does it raise for you?

At the point when you recognize these triggers, you can begin to investigate why they convey such a lot of weight and whether you can lessen their significance. For instance, a Chief may be humiliated to concede that he blows up while examining numbers since he battled in numerical class. Understanding this trigger may be sufficient. Or on the other hand, the President could decide to review the month-to-month outlines in private to stay away from the trigger of Emotions Like every other person is hanging tight for him.

2. Tune into actual side effects

Focus on how you are feeling, including whether you are Emotions Ravenous or tired. These elements can fuel your Emotions and prompt you to unequivocally decipher your Emotions more. On the off chance that you can resolve the hidden issue (for example hunger, depletion), you can change your close-to-home reaction.

3. Consider the story you are telling yourself

Without data, we fill in the spaces with subtleties of our own. Maybe you are Emotiondismissed after you haven't heard from a relative; you accept it on the grounds that they never again care about you.

Before you make these attributions, ask yourself: what different clarifications may be conceivable? In the case of the relative, what else could be happening with them that could prevent them from contacting you? Might they at some point be occupied or debilitated? Might it be said that they are a

Ace your emotions

good-natured individual who frequently neglects to completely finish responsibilities?

BetterUp's Shonna Waters suggests the "very much like me" procedure. Anything that thought process or activity you are doling out to the next individual (there's quite often someone else involved), add "very much like me" as far as possible. It is an approach to advising yourself that you are likewise a blemished person.

4. Participate in sure self-talk

At the point when our Emotions feel overpowering, our self-talk can become pessimistic: "I screwed up once more" or "every other person is so horrendous." Assuming you treat yourself with sympathy, you can supplant a portion of this pessimistic talk with good remarks. Take a stab at empowering yourself by saying "I generally make a good attempt" or "Individuals are doing all that can be expected." This shift can assist with moderating the Emotions we're feeling. You can in any case be disappointed with a circumstance that isn't working however never again need to relegate fault or sum it up past the circumstance.

5. Pursue a decision about how to answer

By and large, we have a decision about how to answer. Assuming that you will generally answer sensations of outrage by attacking individuals, you probably notice the adverse consequence it is having on your connections. You could likewise see that it doesn't feel far better. Or on the other hand, it feels better right now, yet the results are difficult.

Next time you feel outraged or dreadful, perceive that you get to pick how you need to answer. That acknowledgement is strong. As opposed to blowing up, might you at any point

Ace your emotions

attempt an alternate reaction? Is it workable for you to let somebody know that you're Emotionfurious as opposed to talking cruelly to them? Become inquisitive about what will occur assuming you change your reactions. How could you feel? How did the other individual answer?

6. Search for positive Emotions

Individuals normally trait more weight to gloomy Emotions than good ones. This is known as a cynicism predisposition. Pessimistic Emotions , similar to disturb, outrage, and bitterness will generally convey a great deal of weight. Good sentiments, similar to happiness, interest, and appreciation are calmer. Making a propensity for seeing these positive encounters can help strength and prosperity.

7. Search for a specialist

Dealing with our own Emotions can be troublesome. It requires a serious level of mindfulness. While we're struggling, our profound self-guideline starts to endure. In some cases, we really want an accomplice like a specialist who can assist us with mastering better self-guideline abilities. Luckily, there are various remedial arrangements that can assist us with figuring out how to more readily manage our Emotions .

What is a personal guideline problem?

Close-to-home guideline problem is a condition where somebody experiences issues dealing with their sentiments. This powerlessness to enough control Emotions is alluded to as dysregulation. Dysregulation is an unfortunate capacity to deal with close-to-home reactions or keep responses within satisfactory reach.

An individual with a close-to-home guideline problem is bound to encounter sensational changes in mindset. These vacillations thus adversely influence the individual's activities Profound guideline issues can bring about a portion of the accompanying:

Trouble constructing and keeping up with sound connections

Reckless way of behaving

Excessive touchiness

Regular implosions or fits

Explosions of Emotions that are uprooted onto somebody who didn't hurt

Close-to-home guideline problems can likewise go with other emotional well-being issues. Issues like misery, stress, or marginal behavioural condition frequently confound close to the home guideline.

What is DBT?

There are numerous restorative methodologies that can assist with close-to-home guideline issues. These mediations will generally be commonsense in nature and can find lasting success.

One methodology that can assist with close-to-home dysregulation is argumentative social treatment (DBT). DBT is a kind of mental social treatment that looks to distinguish negative reasoning examples. People work with a specialist to supplant these examples with positive social changes.

DBT is a mental reappraisal strategy. It incorporates practices like idea substitution or situational job inversions. In

Ace your emotions

situational job inversions, the individual envisions what is happening according to an alternate point of view. This exercise can assist them with creating compassion and mental adaptability.

One of the drawn-out objectives of persuasive conduct treatment is to further develop trouble resilience. Trouble resistance is the capacity to sit with awkward Emotions , sensations, and encounters. Close-to-home dysregulation frequently comes from a craving to "supersede" the unwanted inclination. Without mindfulness, individuals will generally fall back on self-hurt, substance misuse, and different ways of behaving to get away from the inclination. Building trouble resilience gives a self-improvement tool stash. This typically incorporates self-calming, interruption, and extremist acknowledgement methods. With training, you can figure out how to quiet yourself down.

Section 6

Kids Emotions

Understanding and dealing with Emotions is significant for improvement and prosperity during youth and adolescence. Emotional learning starts early in life, as youngsters find a great many Emotions , and develops as they develop. This point expects to give a superior comprehension of the critical phases of profound turn of events, its effects, interrelated abilities, and the elements that impact close-to-home skills.

Close-to-home capability (EC) is a formative cycle that contains three interrelated skills:

1) Emotion Articulation;

 2) Emotion Information;

 3) Emotion guidelines (i.e., monitoring one's Emotions and adjusting them when vital). Early in life, youngsters as of now show a scope of Emotions in friendly circumstances through non-verbal messages (e.g., giving an embrace, moping). Then, propels in mental improvement permit kids to distinguish their own and others' Emotions , and the conditions that lead to their demeanour. This close to home getting it, thusly, permits youngsters to screen and to change their Emotions to adapt to tough spots.

Youngsters and teens who can comprehend and deal with their Emotions are bound to:

•express Emotions by talking tranquillity or in fitting ways.

•quickly return in the wake of areas of strength for Emotionlike dissatisfaction, disappointment or energy

Ace your emotions

•control motivations

•act fittingly - that is, in manners that don't hurt others, things or themselves.

Furthermore, this is really great for kids since it assists them with learning, making companions, becoming free and that's just the beginning.

Your youngster's capacity to comprehend and deal with Emotions creates after some time. At the point when your kid is youthful, they'll require to assist with grasping Emotions . This for the most part includes perceiving and naming Emotions , which lays the foundation for dealing with Emotions as your kid ages.

As your youngster develops, they'll learn more procedures to deal with their Emotions without your assistance.

It is additionally called close to home guideline to Comprehend and deal with Emotions . It's a significant piece of your kid's self-guideline.

Youngsters under 3 years: creating a language for Emotions

Youngsters experience Emotions before they can utilise words to portray those Emotions . Youngsters additionally comprehend language before they can utilise it themselves. So you can assist your kid with understanding their Emotions by assisting them with creating a 'close to home language.

It could feel peculiar to converse with your kid about sentiments while they're actually creating language abilities. Here are thoughts to help:

At the point when you see your kid showing a specific inclination, name it for themselves and discuss it. For instance, 'You have a major grin all over. You should be glad to see me, or 'You're crying. You're disappointed on the grounds that you can't play with the fish'.

Ace your emotions

Mark the Emotions your kid finds in you and others. For instance, 'Aunt's miserable in light of the fact that she misses Granddad'.

Assist your youngster with investigating Emotions through play. Play thoughts to foster small kids' Emotions incorporate manikin play, singing, perusing and untidy play.

Kids 3-8 years

figuring out how to comprehend and deal with Emotions

Youngsters foster their capacity to perceive and name Emotions through a lot of training. It's simpler for youngsters to rehearse through play, when they're loose, or before their Emotions get excessively serious.

Here are ways you can assist your kid with working on perceiving and naming Emotions :

Discuss the Emotions that characters in books, Television programs or motion pictures may insight. For instance, 'Check Bluey's face out. She looks miserable.

Peruse books about Emotions with your youngster. Most importantly, you could attempt The manner in which I feel by Janan Cain, About sentiments from Usborne, or F is for sentiments by Goldie Millar and Lisa A. Berger.

Show your kid how you perceive your Emotions and assist them with perceiving theirs. For instance, 'When I broke that glass, I shouted actually boisterously. Does that happen to you when you drive a slip-up and feel mad?'

Assist your youngster with working out how their body feels while they're encountering an inclination. For instance, 'You look anxious. Do you have butterflies in your belly?'

Offer your kid chances to investigate Emotions through play. Play thoughts to foster preschooler Emotions   and play thoughts to foster young Emotions incorporate muddled play, drawing or painting, manikin play, moving and music play.

Complete an Emotions movement with your youngster. You pick an inclination like 'invigorated' and act it out with your kid. You can transform this movement into a basic speculating game.

You can likewise begin assisting your kid with learning basic methodologies to deal with their Emotions .

 For instance:

Help your youngster with ways of quieting down major areas of strength from building up to 10 or taking 5 full breaths.

Recommend ways of responding to serious areas of strength for to - for instance, applaud when you're energised, request an embrace when you're miserable, or crush your pad truly hard when you're furious.

Pre-youngsters and teens

fortifying close-to-home abilities

Pre-adolescents and young people frequently have areas of strength for feel in some cases overpowering Emotions like disgrace and embarrassment. They could know the words for these Emotions yet experience difficulty remembering them when they're disturbed. Additionally, as a result of high school mental health, young people don't necessarily have what it takes to communicate and deal with Emotions in a grown-up manner.

That is the reason pre-adolescent young people actually need assistance with understanding and dealing with Emotions . With training, your kid will actually want to deal with their Emotions without you.

Ace your emotions

Here are thoughts to fortify your youngster's capacity to comprehend and deal with Emotions in the adolescent years:

Step in when you can see Emotions developing. The sooner your youngster can recognize their profound changes, the more straightforward it will be for them to remain in charge of their way of behaving.

Assist your kid with seeing early actual indications of compelling Emotions . For instance, 'When I was stranded in rush hour gridlock yesterday, my heart was hustling and I felt truly hot. Does that happen to you when you're baffled?'

Assist your kid with seeing early conduct indications of compelling Emotions . For instance, 'You're beginning to hit that console a piece hard. Do you have to stop briefly and get some outside air?'

Talk with your kid about what you do when you notice the signs and areas of strength that are developing. For instance, 'When I begin to feel truly furious with myself, I centre around something I'm truly glad for all things considered. Could that work for you?'

Work with your kid on a rundown of things they could do when they notice compelling Emotions developing, such as going for a run, paying attention to noisy music on their earphones, or reflecting.

Attempt to incorporate a lot of choices so your kid can pick ones that vibe right in various circumstances.

Recollect that consulting with youngsters about Emotions will not be as viable while they're battling with serious areas of strength. You really want to step in ahead of schedule or hold on until the inclination has passed.

Signs your youngster could require help to deal with their Emotions

Ace your emotions

All youngsters need assistance and support in areas of strength to oversee some of the time, particularly more youthful kids or youngsters managing additional difficulties like passing in the family or other horrendous mishaps.

Youngsters could require help with major areas of strength for overseeing on the off chance that they have a bombshell or hopeless outlook on how overpowering their Emotions are

feel areas of strength for exceptionally that is messed up with regards to the issue or circumstance

still areas of strength for a feel for quite a while after whatever ignited the Emotions

frequently go from being quiet to Emotional extreme inclination like indignation rapidly

express Emotions improperly - for instance, chuckling in light of terrible news

go extremely calm, stow away or drive individuals away when they're overpowered.

Additionally, pre-high schoolers and teen kids could require help if they:

appear to settle on unfortunate choices since they feel compelling Emotions like disappointment

find it hard to loosen up to the point of partaking in their leisure activities or accompanying loved ones.

Advantages of assisting your youngsters with figuring out Emotions

Very much like grown-ups, kids need to foster procedures for dealing with their Emotions , so they can assemble social-profound abilities. At the point when youngsters are all the more socially and sincerely mindful and gifted, they can

Ace your emotions

all the more successfully explore connections, quiet down and issue settle when difficulties emerge.

At the point when parental figures have prevailed with regards to directing themselves, they can relate to the youngster's close-to-home insight and ponder it, instead of attempting to "fix" the inclination. For instance, a grown-up could say, "Aw, you're making some intense memories, right? I know it's truly baffling when you would rather not leave the jungle gym." Later, when the kid has quieted down, the grown-up can direct the kid's way of behaving or help the kid's issue settle, for instance by saying, "I realise you blow up when we leave the jungle gym, however, you can't hit me. How might we make it more straightforward when we need to leave?"

With a baby, the reaction ought to be less verbal - it's more about the parental figure's manner of speaking, non-verbal communication, and even relaxation. Furthermore, it typically implies remaining truly near the youngster.

"Indeed, even a furious kid will in any case need you close by to give an Emotion Of safety," Havighurst says.

It's likewise essential to give your very best to plan for troublesome minutes, she says. One major piece is taking care of oneself. "It's not unexpected what comes last when you have small kids," she says. "Be that as it may, it's difficult to be sincerely in a decent space to comprehend and manage your own Emotions assuming that you are totally stripped."

Understanding what your own programmed reactions are is fundamental also - and having the apparatuses set up to hinder them. At the point when we're set off, we frequently go into a "battle, flight, freeze" reaction that we can't think right out of. All things being equal, we really want to have a few procedures set up that includes our actual body and sensory

Ace your emotions

system, like breathing or extending. We likewise need to rehearse them ahead of time so that, in an extreme second, they're readily available.

The language of individuals who raise you and their approaches to answering Emotions become incorporated as your own discourse," Havighurst says. "Guardians are the cerebrum, or the controller, for exceptionally small kids more often than not."

A youngster who is disregarded or raged at for having specific sentiments might figure out how to keep away from or stifle them. Yet, in the event that a parental figure has figured out how to be agreeable enough with Emotions to remain with youngsters during a troublesome second and let them in on they are protected and cherished regardless of what they are feeling, the kids will generally foster better survival strategies, Havighurst says. Kids with uneasiness are bound to have guardians who are cavalier of Emotions - which could mostly make sense of why emotional training might diminish small kids' tension.

This approach might appear to be extremist to the individuals who have been instructed that a kid who cries or pitches a fit ought to be overlooked or even rebuffed. However, specialists highlight that it's anything but a question of being tolerant. All things being equal, it is tied in with keeping up with limits in a compassionate, yet firm, way. In the long haul, emotion training is intended to help kids through extreme minutes with the goal that they are at last better ready to direct themselves. It is likewise a question of needs. Many guardians go through hours helping their kids to ride a bike or present the letter set. The close-to-home ability has been connected in adulthood to better mental and actual well-being, more grounded

Ace your emotions

connections, and even work execution. Given its significance to such countless parts of our lives, the inquiry isn't the reason we would invest energy and work to beat our own distress to assist our youngsters with figuring out how to comprehend, acknowledge, and suitably express their sentiments. The genuine inquiry is,Grasping Youngsters' Emotions .

The capacity to appreciate people at their core isn't fixed. Youngsters can figure out how to distinguish and perceive their Emotions and pick how they wish to answer what is going on.

Discussing their sentiments

Discussing sentiments and communicating Emotions can assist with dealing with Emotions and give fundamental new points of view.

Looking for help

Requesting help is a strength, not a shortcoming. While autonomy is great, it can prompt passing up learning.

Three stages for fostering the propensity include:

•Perceive when to request help.

•Realise the kind of help required.

•Ask the perfect individual for help.

Showing great habits

It tends to be valuable to talk about what great habits could resemble with the kid. All things considered, there are numerous social subtleties and varying degrees of assumption in light of the climate.

By gaining what they anticipate from others, it can assist them with dealing with their Emotions and coming about conduct.

Attempting new things

Ace your emotions

While helpful for physical and psychological wellness, getting out of their usual range of familiarity can likewise be a significant approach to acquiring certainty and more noteworthy command over how youngsters think and act.

Figuring out how to share

It very well may be an effective approach to distinguishing and rehearsing a cooperative way of behaving.

Conquering conflicts under the surface

Youngsters might find it valuable to contrast how they now feel battling and emotion versus how they would feel in the event that their reasoning changed. Utilise the three stages in Within and Outside exercise to comprehend How would I think? Feel? Also, what do I do?

Eliminating the veils

Youngsters, similar to grown-ups, frequently veil how they feel. Utilise the Inclination Veils practise with kids to assist them with perceiving what kind of cover they put on when they would rather not manage something they feel.

The basic demonstration of discussing Emotions with youngsters can help them distinguish and name their sentiments and comprehend that they control how they respond to circumstances.

Ace your emotions

Section 7

Poor profound well-being can debilitate your body's insusceptible framework.

This makes you bound to get colds and different diseases during sincerely troublesome times. Likewise, when you are Emotions Worried, restless, or upset, you may not deal with your well-being as well as you should. Good profound well-being begins with monitoring your considerations, sentiments, and ways of behaving. Learning solid ways of adapting to pressure and issues is an ordinary piece of life. Having a decent outlook on yourself is critical to have sound connections.

Numerous things that occur in your life can disturb your profound well-being. These can prompt overwhelming inclinations of trouble, stress, or nervousness. Indeed, even great or needed changes can be essentially as distressing as undesirable changes. These things include:

•A pandemic

•Being laid off from your work.

•Having a kid leave or get back.

•Managing the demise of a friend or family member.

•Getting separated or hitched.

•Experiencing an ailment or a physical issue.

•Finding a new line of work advancement.

•Encountering cash issues.

•Moving to another home.

•Having or taking on a child.

Your body answers the manner in which you think, feel, and act. This is one sort of "mind/body association." When you are worried, restless, or upset, your body responds truly. For instance, you could foster hypertension or a stomach ulcer after an especially unpleasant occasion, like the demise of a friend or family member.

While emotional well-being issue in the working environment may constantly be available somewhat, it is preventable by and large from happening by any means or basically decreased in their effect through Advancement, Avoidance and Early Mediation (PPEI). The critical components of a viable methodology for counteraction are the accompanying:

Building all-encompassing mindfulness for the individual, the authority and the association

Recognizing issues at the beginning phase and seeing the patterns of people and groups

Building a believed encouraging group of people to address difficulties before they become issues

Registration all the more consistently and offering welcomed help to those under strain in the period of scarcity

Making a mentally protected culture where it is alright to be a powerless and welcome help.

Profound Heartbeat was created during the Covid pandemic to mitigate the test individuals experienced around psychological well-being and how telecommuting decreased individuals' capacity to register and back each other during seasons of strain.

The innovation is an underlying arrangement with viable emotional well-being structures of advancement, anticipation and early mediation support. Support is best when is it ideal, welcomed, trusted and talented. Profound Heartbeat cultivates this sort of help in a reasonable, private and human way, where innovation improves human empathic associations.

Ace your emotions

We are decreasing the disgrace connected with psychological wellness, expanding close-to-home mindfulness and successful help that forestalls ongoing psychological well-being issues.

Way to Further developed Wellbeing

There are ways of working on your close-to-home well-being. To start with, perceive your Emotions and comprehend the reason why you are having them. Figuring out the reasons for trouble, stress, and nervousness in your life can assist you with dealing with your profound well-being. Following are a few other supportive tips.

Express your sentiments in proper ways.

On the off chance that sensations of stress, misery, or tension are creating actual issues, keeping these sentiments inside can aggravate you. It's alright to tell your friends and family when something is irritating you. In any case, remember that your loved ones may not generally have the option to assist you with managing your sentiments fittingly. At these times, ask somebody outside the circumstance for help. Have a go at asking your family specialist, an instructor, or a strict consultant for counsel and backing to assist you with working on your profound well-being.

Carry on with a healthy lifestyle.

Centre around the things that you are thankful for in your life. Do whatever it takes not to fixate on the issues at work, school, or home that lead to gloomy sentiments. This doesn't mean you need to claim to be content when you feel worried, restless, or upset. It's critical to manage gloomy sentiments yet attempt to zero in on the positive things in your day-to-day existence, as well. You might need to utilise a diary to monitor things that cause you to feel blissful or quiet. Some

Ace your emotions

examinations have shown that having an uplifting perspective can work on your personal satisfaction and give your well-being a lift. You may likewise have to track down ways of relinquishing a few things in your day-to-day existence that cause you to feel worried and overpowered. Set aside a few minutes for things you appreciate.

Foster strength.

Individuals with strength are better at adapting to pressure in a sound manner. Versatility can be learned and fortified with various techniques. These incorporate having social help, keeping a positive perspective on yourself, tolerating change, and keeping things in context. An instructor or specialist can assist you with accomplishing this objective with mental social treatment.

Deal with yourself.

To have great close-to-home well-being, it's vital to deal with your body by having a standard daily practice. This incorporates an everyday practice of quality feasts, rest, and exercise to ease repressed pressure. Try not to gorge and don't manhandle medications or liquor. Utilising medications or liquor noble motivations different issues, like family and medical conditions

Quiet your brain and body.

Unwinding strategies, for example, contemplation, paying attention to music, paying attention to directed symbolism tracks, yoga, and Kendo are valuable ways of bringing your Emotions into balance.

Reflection is a type of directed thought. It can take many structures. For instance, you might do it by working out, extending, or breathing profoundly. Ask your family specialist for an exhortation about unwinding techniques.

Ace your emotions

Interesting points

Poor close-to-home well-being can debilitate your body's safe framework. This makes you bound to get colds and different diseases during genuinely troublesome times. Likewise, when you are Emotions Worried, restless, or upset, you may not deal with your well-being as well as you ought to. You may not want to work out, eat nutritious food sources, or take medication that your primary care physician endorses. You might manhandle liquor, tobacco, or different medications. Different indications of poor close-to-home well-being incorporate

back torment

change in hunger

chest torment

clogging or the runs

dry mouth

outrageous sluggishness

general a throbbing painfulness

migraines

hypertension

sleep deprivation (inconvenience resting)

wooziness

palpitations (the inclination that your heart is hustling)

sexual issues

windedness

firm neck

perspiring

resentful stomach

weight gain or misfortune

Ace your emotions

how accomplishes profound heartbeat work

Individuals log their profound state on their gadget at a picked recurrence and time

Programming gives bits of knowledge to people and groups about profound examples

People with patterns pushing toward risk zones are made mindful and urged to welcome help

Individuals in danger can self-right and recurrence of checks-in increments until they are protected

Protection of people is kept up consistently until they decide to welcome confided-in help

Group patterns of close-to-home heartbeat are given to pioneers of mindfulness and culture upgrades

Section 8

Positive reaction/vibe

At the point when our minds go negative, that can consume our efficiency, inventiveness, and thinking abilities. That is because negative considerations will generally have a greater effect than positive contemplations. Once more, this returns to development. Endurance relied upon having the option to identify and stay away from risky circumstances.

Moulding your brain to encounter more sure

Energy doesn't necessarily allude to just grinning and looking lively, but — inspiration is more around one's general viewpoint on life and their propensity to zero in on generally what is great throughout everyday life.

In this piece, we'll cover the fundamentals of energy inside certain brain science, recognize a portion of the many advantages of moving toward life according to a positive perspective, and investigate a few hints and methods for developing a positive outlook.

This piece is a long one, so get comfortable and settle in.

Before you read on, we figured you could get a kick out of the chance to download our three Positive Brain science Activities free of charge. These science-based activities will investigate essential parts of positive brain research including qualities, values and self-sympathy and will give you the instruments to upgrade the prosperity of your clients, understudies or employees. You presumably have a thought of what a positive outlook or inspirational perspective is as of now, yet it's dependably useful, to begin with, a definition.

"Positive reasoning is a psychological and close-to-home mentality that spotlights the brilliant side of life and anticipates positive outcomes."

Positive reasoning implies moving toward life's difficulties with an uplifting perspective. It doesn't guarantee to mean staying away from or overlooking the terrible things; all things being equal, it includes capitalising on the possibly terrible circumstances, attempting to see the best in others, and surveying yourself and your capacities in a positive light."

We can extrapolate from these definitions and concoct a decent portrayal of a positive mentality as the inclination to zero in on the splendid side, anticipate positive outcomes, and move toward difficulties with an uplifting perspective.

Having a positive mentality implies regularly practising positive reasoning, ceaselessly looking for the silver lining and making the best out of any circumstance you regard yourself as in.

Qualities and Characteristics of a Positive Outlook:

All in all, presently we understand what a positive outlook would we say it is, and can plunge into the following significant inquiry: What does it resemble?

There are numerous qualities and qualities related to a positive outlook, including:

Good faith: an eagerness to try and take a risk as opposed to expecting your endeavours won't pay off.

Acknowledgement: recognizing that things don't necessarily in all cases turn out how you need them to, yet gaining from your errors.

Ace your emotions

Flexibility: quickly returning from misfortune, frustration, and disappointment as opposed to surrendering.

Appreciation: effectively, and consistently valuing the beneficial things in your day-to-day existence.

Cognizance/Care: devoting the psyche to cognizant mindfulness and upgrading the capacity to centre.

Honesty: the quality of being noteworthy, noble, and clear, rather than underhanded and self-serving Not exclusively are these qualities of a positive outlook, but they may likewise work in the other direction — effectively taking on idealism, acknowledgement, versatility, appreciation, care, and respectability in your life will help you create and keep a positive mentality.

A Rundown of Inspirational perspectives

On the off chance that you found the rundown above still excessively dubious, there are a lot more unambiguous instances of an uplifting outlook in real life.

For instance, inspirational perspectives can include:

It is looking at affliction without flinching… and snickering.

•Getting what you get, and not throwing a tantrum.

•Partaking in the unforeseen, in any event, when it's not what you needed initially.

•Spurring people around you with a positive word.

•Utilising the force of a grin to switch the tone of a circumstance.

•Being agreeable to those you don't have any idea.

It's getting back up when you tumble down. (Regardless of how frequently you tumble down.)

•Being a wellspring of energy that lifts people around you.

•Understanding that connections are a higher priority than material things.

Ace your emotions

•Being blissful in any event, when you have nearly nothing.

•Living it up in any event, when you are losing.

•Being glad for another person's prosperity.

•Having a positive future vision, regardless of how terrible your ongoing conditions are.

•Grinning.

•Giving a pat on the back, even to a complete outsider.

•Tell somebody you realise that they worked effectively.

•Filling somebody's heart with joy. (In addition to a kid's… grown-ups prefer to have their day be unique, as well!)

It's not whining regardless of how out-of-line things give off an impression of being. (It is an exercise in futility… all things considered, follow through with something!)

•Not allowing others' cynicism to cut you down.

•Offering more than you hope to get as a trade-off.

•Being reliable with yourself…

Presently we discover somewhat more about what a positive outlook resembles, we can go to one of the greatest inquiries of all:

What's going on with having an uplifting perspective?

What is it about having a positive mentality that is so significant, so effective, so extraordinary?

Indeed, the qualities and attributes recorded above give us a clue; in the event that you go over the writing, you'll see plenty of advantages connected to hopefulness, versatility, and care.

You'll see that mindfulness and uprightness are connected to better personal satisfaction, and acknowledgement and appreciation can take you from the "OK life" to the "easy street."

The Significance of Fostering the Right Contemplations

Ace your emotions

Fostering a genuinely sure outlook and acquiring these advantages is a component of the considerations you develop.

You can definitely relax — this piece isn't about the sort of certain reasoning that is all sure, constantly. We don't guarantee that just "figuring cheerful contemplations" will present to you all the achievements you want throughout everyday life, and we unquestionably don't completely accept that idealism is justified in each circumstance, all day long.

Fostering the right contemplations isn't tied in with being continually blissful or happy, and there's really no need to focus on overlooking anything negative or unsavoury in your life. It's tied in with integrating both the positive and negative into your point of view and deciding to in any case be for the most part hopeful.

It's tied in with recognizing that you won't generally be blissful and figuring out how to acknowledge awful states of mind and troublesome Emotions when they come.

Most importantly, it's tied in with expanding your command over your own disposition despite whatever comes in your direction. You have zero control over your temperament, and you can't necessarily control the considerations that jump into your head, yet you can pick how you handle them.

At the point when you decide to surrender to the cynicism, negativity, and pessimism perspective on the world, you are not just submitting to a deficiency of control and possibly floundering in misery — you are passing up a significant chance for development and improvement.

As per positive clinician Barbara Fredrickson, pessimistic reasoning, and gloomy Emotions have their place: they permit you to hone your emphasis on risks, dangers, and weaknesses. This is fundamental for endurance, albeit maybe not however much it was for our precursors.

Then again, positive reasoning and positive Emotions "expand and construct" our assets and abilities, and free us up to conceivable outcomes.

Building a positive structure for your viewpoints isn't tied in with being effervescent and annoyingly bright, but making an interest in yourself and your future. It's alright to feel down or think cynically at times, yet deciding to answer with good faith, strength, and appreciation will help you undeniably more over the long haul.

Assume command over the things you can, and acknowledge the things you can't. Remind yourself "Never a disappointment, consistently an illustration;" make each disappointment a learning a valuable open door. Attempt the mirror method — praise yourself (and really mean it) each time you see yourself in the mirror. To be hopeful, you need to change what you understand with regard to yourself and the circumstance you are experiencing. Positive convictions bring about a more certain result, which then, at that point, prompts a more uplifting perspective.

The Results of an Inspirational perspective

Besides upgrading your abilities and individual assets, there are numerous different advantages of developing a positive mentality, including better general well-being, better capacity to adapt to pressure, and more prominent prosperity.

As indicated by specialists positive reasoning can expand your life expectancy, lessen paces of despondency and levels of pain, give you more prominent protection from the normal cold, further develop your general mental and actual prosperity, work on your cardiovascular well-being and

Ace your emotions

safeguard you from cardiovascular sickness, and assist you with building adapting abilities to keep you above water during testing times.

You've likely known about this multitude of conventional advantages previously, so we'll get more unambiguous and investigate the advantages of a positive outlook in a few changed settings:

The working environment

Administration

Managing incapacity (for both those with a handicap and people around them)

Nursing and medical services

Recuperation from malignant growth

Advantages of a Positive Mental Disposition in the Work environment

No development better catches the quintessence of an uplifting outlook in the work environment very like mental capital (or PsyCap for short). This multi-component development is comprised of four mental assets:

•Trust

•Adequacy

•Flexibility

•Positive thinking

•PsyCap was emphatically connected with work fulfilment, hierarchical responsibility, and mental prosperity.

Ace your emotions

•PsyCap was additionally decidedly connected with hierarchical citizenship (beneficial worker ways of behaving) and different proportions of execution (self-appraised, manager assessments, and goal measures).

•PsyCap was adversely connected with pessimism, turnover goals, work pressure, and nervousness.

PsyCap was likewise adversely connected with negative representative abnormality.

It appears to be really direct that uplifting perspectives like hopefulness and strength lead to positive results for the association and for the representatives!

One more concentrate by a couple of the monsters in the field of positive brain science explored the connection between bliss and advantages to representatives. They showed that uplifting outlooks in the working environment likewise benefit the representative notwithstanding the association:

More joyful representatives are more useful than different workers.

Blissful sales reps have higher deals than different sales reps.

Blissful workers are more imaginative than different representatives.

Cheerful representatives are assessed all the more decidedly by their bosses.

Cheerful workers are more averse to showing work withdrawal (non-appearance, turnover, work burnout, and retaliatory ways of behaving).

Cheerful workers get more cash flow than different representatives.

All in this way, an uplifting outlook can have extraordinary advantages for the association all in all and its workers.

Ace your emotions

It just so happens, an uplifting perspective can likewise bring about benefits for pioneers and their devotees (as well as spreading energy all through the association).

train your cerebrum to turn out to be more sure through these procedures.

1. Notice your contemplations.
The primary spot to begin is by noticing your contemplations - regardless of whether it's only for 10 minutes. Since we're animals of propensities, you might see that you have similar negative contemplations sneaking up on you. Could it be said that you are restless about a forthcoming excursion? Are worried about work? Are you annoyed about that battle you had with your spouse? Once you understand what negative considerations are irritating you the most, you can begin chipping away at an answer for resolving the issue. For instance, on the off chance that you're truly irritated by a collaborator, move toward your supervisor with the issue and inquire as to whether you can be moved to one more piece of the workplace where you don't need to interface with them as much. Once you understand what negative contemplations are annoying you the most, you can begin dealing with an answer to resolve the issue. For instance, in the event that you're truly irritated by a colleague, move toward your manager with the issue and inquire as to whether you can be moved to one more

piece of the workplace where you don't need to collaborate with them so much.

2. Examine the 3 everyday upsides.

Before you fall asleep you can undoubtedly prepare your mind. Ponder your day and contemplate three explicit beneficial things that happened to you that day. Whether in the event that it was somebody getting you some espresso, an incredibly gorgeous nightfall, or handling another client. Indeed, even the littlest things, such as being given a pat on the back, eating with a close buddy, or watching your canine roll around, are all that could possibly be needed to fulfil you

3. Give somebody a whoop.

Appreciation is truly significant. Research has found that showing appreciation can do anything from making you more hopeful to warding off coronary supply route sickness. An appreciation diary is a decent spot to begin, yet I've observed that sharing your appreciation is undeniably more valuable

4. Encircle yourself with positive individuals.

Since Emotions are infectious, it just seems OK that you would need to encircle yourself with good individuals who rouse, engage, and inspire you

5.. Care for your body and brain.

Research has figured out endlessly opportunity again that dealing with ourselves actually and intellectually can impact our satisfaction and train our cerebrum over the long run to be more certain.

6. Subconscious re-preparing and inward mending.

Now and again to turn out to be more certain, we need to reveal and afterwards discharge the previous negative encounters that we've been clutching. Practices like tapping, day-to-day assertions, neuro-etymological programming, and

Ace your emotions

mirror work can help you find and mend these injuries. Furthermore, these activities can assist you with building a more steady and certifying conviction framework that you can utilise the following time you face any horrendous encounters.

Positive Encounters

The Positive Encounters worksheet is a basic one in principle, yet it tends to be challenging to finish in fact. The trouble accompanies an identical prize, however; you can get an extraordinary lift in your temperament, confidence, and fearlessness from finishing it.

The main guidance is to think about every one of the positive characteristics recorded and expound momentarily on times when you have shown every one of them.

The positive characteristics include:

Fortitude

Generosity

Benevolence

Love

Penance

Shrewdness

Joy

Assurance

Assuming you're Emotionespecially down, you might be enticed to avoid a couple, yet battle this desire! You have most certainly shown every one of these qualities all at once or another — don't undercut yourself!

1.Positive Moves toward Prosperity

This asset is really a freebie, however, you can surely make it intuitive by taking notes or utilising marks to demonstrate what you have attempted, or what you might want to try

These exercises advance positive

Being caring to yourself

Work-out consistently

Take up a side interest or potentially become familiar with another expertise

Have some good times

Be careful with beverages and medications

See the master plan

Tolerating: "It is for all intents and purposes"

To peruse more about how every one of these exercises adds to your prosperity, download the gift here.

Positive   Self-Talk/Adapting Considerations Worksheet

The positive self-talk/adapting considerations worksheet is an extraordinary method for diverting your concentration from the negative to the positive and concocting positive explanations you can use to adapt in future distressing or tough spots.

Model adapting considerations and positive proclamations recorded on the worksheet include:

Stop, and inhale, I can do this.

This will pass.

This feels terrible, and sentiments are regularly off-base.

I can feel terrible yet decide to take a new and sound course.

I feel as such on account of my previous encounters, however, I'm protected at the present time.

Ace your emotions

Subsequent to perusing the model assertions, the worksheet urges you to record some adapting considerations or positive explanations for troublesome or upsetting circumstances in your day-to-day existence. You can think of them straightforwardly on the worksheet, yet it could be generally useful to duplicate them onto a note card and convey them to you.

We have various Emotions and considerations, and we have such a wide assortment which is as it should be. Times while being a piece critical can help us, and it is smart to let out the gloomy Emotions you experience sometimes (particularly in the event that the option is restraining them).

Assuming you're a hopeful person naturally, develop an appreciation for your intrinsic energy, yet ensure you don't shove aside the pessimistic sentiments that yield up. They're essential for life as well.

On the off chance that you're a worry wart naturally, don't surrender all expectations regarding truly thinking decidedly. Attempt a couple of the strategies that appear to be generally relevant and offer yourself a reprieve in the event that it requires some investment. Keep in mind, the objective isn't to turn into a "Pollyanna," but to turn into the best self that you can be and keep a sound and cheerful mental state.

Section 9

Craft of consideration

Really great for the psyche

Being caring lifts serotonin and dopamine, which are synapses in the cerebrum that give you sensations of fulfilment and prosperity, and cause the joy/reward to focus in your mind. Endorphins, which are your body's normal pain reliever, likewise can be delivered

"Research offers that grace is the area of strength for a lively social commitment, which thusly is a basic part of generally cerebrum wellbeing."

To decide what graciousness means for cerebrum wellbeing, the group requested that guardians review their own strengths and report on their children's sympathy during the preparation program.

They observed that guardians are stronger and preschoolers are more compassionate after benevolence preparation. Both versatility and sympathy require mental abilities like answering great to stressors or taking into account alternate points of view.

Their discoveries thus support the possibility that generosity can impact mental capability and by and large mind well-being.

Shockingly, the specialists found that kids' compassion levels stayed sub-optimal regardless of the recognizable improvement in the wake of preparation. This may be on the grounds that Coronavirus well-being estimates essentially restricted children's typical social and close-to-home learning.

The analysts likewise tried whether understanding the science behind the consideration-preparing program influences guardians' versatility

Guardians can learn basic methodologies for rehearsing benevolence successfully, squarely in their own homes, to establish a mind-sound climate for their children. "In the midst of stress, pausing for a minute to rehearse graciousness for you and model it for your kids can support your own flexibility and further develop your kid's prosocial ways of behaving," said Fratantoni.

"Try not to misjudge the force of consideration, since it can eventually change and shape cerebrum wellbeing."

The effects of benevolence might try and stretch out past families. "Thoughtfulness can be a strong mind well-being sponsor that raises flexibility, for guardians and families, yet for society in general," said Johnson.

Investigating Thoughtfulness as a Potentiator for Improved Cerebrum Wellbeing

A developing group of exploration has proposed that elevated degrees of family working — frequently estimated as sure parent-kid correspondence and low degrees of parental pressure — are related to a more grounded mental turn of events, more elevated levels of school commitment, and more fruitful friend relations as youth age.

The Coronavirus pandemic has carried colossal interruption to different parts of day-to-day existence, particularly for guardians of small kids, ages 3-5, who face disengagement, separation, and extraordinary changes to how they draw in

Ace your emotions

and mingle. Luckily, both youth and parent minds are plastic and responsive to change.

Flexibility research shows that elements like participating in thoughtful gestures, creating confiding in connections, and answering mercifully to the sensations of others can help lay new brain processes and work on personal satisfaction. However, little exploration has examined the impacts of cerebrum-sound parental acts of generosity with pre-school mature kids.

The ongoing review looks at whether an intelligent, parent-youngster generosity educational program can act as a potentiator for mental well-being as estimated by flexibility and kid sympathy levels.

During the pinnacle of the pandemic, mother members between the ages of 26-46 (n = 38, finish rate 75%) finished polls on parental versatility levels and parent-detailed youngster empathic support of social ways of behaving when taking part in a month on the web, independent, generosity educational plan.

A big part of the gathering got extra mind well-being schooling making sense of the standards of brain adaptability, sympathy, point of view taking, and versatility. Moms in the two gatherings showed expanded strength (p < 0.001) and revealed more significant levels of empathic conduct in their youngsters (p < 0.001) subsequent to finishing the educational program.

There was no massive contrast between gatherings. Examination of mean flexibility levels during Coronavirus to pre-pandemic general means showed that moms are announcing fundamentally lower levels of strength as well as diminished sympathetic ways of behaving in their youngsters.

Ace your emotions

These outcomes support the thought that benevolence is a strong mind well-being sponsor that can build versatility and sympathy.

This examination study was convenient and pertinent for guardians considering the heap of stresses achieved by the continuous Coronavirus pandemic. There are more extensive general well-being suggestions for outfitting people with devices to adopt a proactive and protection strategy for their cerebrum wellbeing.

Balance Your Psychological And Profound Wellbeing

Liberality is more than direct. The speciality of thoughtfulness implies holding onto an emotional supportiveness, as well as being liberal and chivalrous, and doing as such without anticipating anything consequently. Thoughtfulness is the nature of being. The demonstration of giving thoughtfulness frequently is sans basic, positive and solid.

Great for the body

Generosity has been displayed to increment confidence, sympathy and empathy, and further develop temperament. It can diminish pulse and cortisol, a pressure chemical, which straightforwardly influences Emotions of anxiety. Individuals who give of themselves in a reasonable manner likewise will generally be better and live longer. Graciousness can build your emotional network with others, which can straightforwardly affect forlornness, work on a low mindset and improve connections overall. It likewise can be infectious.

Ace your emotions

Searching for ways of offering grace can give you a centre action, particularly on the off chance that you will generally be restless or focused in a few social circumstances.

Really great for the brain

Physiologically, thoughtfulness can decidedly change your cerebrum. Being thoughtful lifts serotonin and dopamine, which are synapses in the cerebrum that give you sensations of fulfilment and prosperity, and cause the delight/reward focuses in your mind to illuminate. Endorphins, which are your body's normal pain reliever, additionally can be delivered. Find ways you can make joy.

Be caring to yourself

It isn't exactly the way that you treat others — it is the means by which you broaden those equivalent ways of behaving and goals to yourself too. I accept you can be kinder in your own self-talk and practice appreciation. Individuals are great at verbally pounding themselves and seldom accomplish that work as a motivational speech. Rather, cynicism frequently makes you disentangle and may try and make an endless loop of consistently getting down on yourself. You wouldn't converse with your neighbour in the manner in which you some of the time converse with yourself. This is the very thing I call the "great neighbour strategy," which can be useful. In the event that you wouldn't agree that it to your great neighbour, don't express it about yourself.

Make a move

Basically inquiring "How am I going to rehearse consideration today?" can be useful. For a schoolwork task, I have welcomed a few clients to focus and occasionally report during the day their proof of consideration to other people and particularly to themselves. This positive centre resembles

Ace your emotions

sowing positive seeds in your brain garden. Where the centre goes, energy streams.

I as of late was discussing benevolence with a youthful client who inquired as to whether I maintained that they should get on the ark. I asked what that implied. The client expressed, "Demonstrations of irregular graciousness." That was an extraordinary reaction from a youngster. What about you? Is it safe to say that you will get on the ark?

Assisting an older individual with a task, chipping in a soup kitchen, surrendering your seat in the transport, or paying for a more unusual espresso are a couple of thoughtful gestures you might have offered or gotten in your life. Thoughtfulness feels better, whether you are the beneficiary or the practitioner. Your mind receives the rewards of generosity as well. This World Thoughtfulness Day, find out about how generosity can make you live longer, better, and more joyful

Benevolence advances a long and sound life

The study of consideration uncovers that being caring can assist you with living better for longer. It was found that the people who participated in chipping-in exercises had lower provocative mixtures than the individuals who didn't . This additionally features the significance of graciousness to oneself. Being self-caring and kind to yourself likewise diminishes provocative mixtures

Thoughtfulness towards your family, companions, and individuals around you advance sound social associations. Studies affecting the north of 300,000 individuals detailed that those with solid social connections are half bound to carry on with a more extended life. Positive social associations further develop pressure reactions and help in laying out sound ways of behaving.

Ace your emotions

Thoughtfulness helps you de-stress

Stress is related to many negative well-being results. You can peruse more about the effect of weight on the cerebrum here. Being thoughtful makes positive and strong associations and satisfies a fundamental requirement for empathy. Along these lines, it can cushion pressure. Very much like wearing defensive gear while cycling supports the effect of falls, irregular thoughtful gestures cushion the pressure of daily existence. North of 300 members who were prepared to be more caring as a pressure decrease procedure, found that their pressure chemical, cortisol, diminished by 51% thus .Cortisol levels should be kept up with low sums for ideal cerebrum working.

Graciousness makes you more joyful

It is acknowledged that being benevolent and liberal feels far better. Cerebrum sweeps of individuals who involved their cash to help others showed more prominent action in mind regions engaged with joy These individuals likewise announced Emotionmore joy after the gift. Members doled out to perform 3 thoughtful gestures once every day for a considerable length of time revealed an expansion in sure temperament Satisfaction experienced was higher when the thoughtful gesture was self-spurred, Fulfilling the necessities of commonality, skill, and self-inspiration works on mental prosperity. Aiding a companion (commonality) may likewise include critical time spent together. Being adequately skilful to help and oneself inspired choice to assist with satisfying the requirements for ideal inspirational impact. Being benevolent and framing a positive social association likewise delivers oxytocin (additionally called love chemical), which increments dopamine creation.

Ace your emotions

Benevolence gives you "assistant's high"

Benevolence enacts your dopamine framework, the prize and joy framework that is actuated by great food and pleasurable exercises. Mind imaging showed that giving cash enacted the dopamine framework, adding to the vibe great "high" experienced after a caring deed. Dopamine is additionally associated with managing inspiration, in this way reassuring proceeded with thoughtful gestures. In a fascinating review, a prescription that increments dopamine levels in the mind was given to members prior to being approached to part cash among themselves and an outsider. Those that were cured showed more generosity and were bound to part the cash similarly

Benevolence diminishes tension

Being caring can likewise assist with diminishing the sensations of social tension. Restless members taking part in thoughtful gestures for quite a long time detailed perking up and diminish in uneasiness side effects. Indeed, even inside thinking kind contemplations and wishing individuals well in friendly circumstances assist with bringing down tension. Working on friendly association and expansion in feel-great mind synthetics can add to this impact.

Being benevolent is a straightforward and powerful method for emotions significantly improved. This November thirteenth, on World Graciousness Day, put forth a cognizant attempt to be more kind to other people and to yourself. Your cerebrum will be much obliged.

The most effective method to Remain mentally collected in Distressing Circumstances — This is What to Do

Stress and emotional well-being are connected. Peruse ways of delivering pressure, including involving green tea to stress the board

Discontinuous fasting for psychological wellness advantages of fasting irregular fasting proof fasting for cerebrum wellbeing

Irregular fasting for emotional wellness benefits: Reality or Craze?

What you eat impacts your cerebrum well-being. The energising proof that proposes that your feast timings can also...

care for psychological wellness cerebrum advantages of careful contemplation care and emotional well-being appreciation and psychological well-being consideration and psychological wellness

Practice benevolence, appreciation, and care for psychological well-being

Learn about how you and your friends and family can feel more joyful on the current year's Worldwide Bliss Day. Look into proof-based strategies to rehearse care, generosity, and appreciation really.

advantages of cold water inundation cold showers for uneasiness cold water treatment benefits emotional wellness cold water dopamine cold shower psychological well-being

Ace your emotions

Finally

Understanding, communicating and adapting to your Emotions can be troublesome, but carving out the opportunity to consider your Emotions , implies you have previously begun to acquire a superior control and comprehension of them.

Utilise the devices referenced in this segment to help yourself and understand that adapting to Emotions isn't simply where we show up and remain - it's a continuous excursion which becomes simpler with time!

Sentiments are only sometimes precise. They are unfortunate perceivers. They can get to a specific measure of truth, yet billows of Emotions frequently obscure reality. Sentiments are planned as a last-option activity or response after the psyche has come to an end result. Sentiments shouldn't go about as a lead or a perceiver. Substantially less, they are not to be empowered to choose a last end. Emotions are there to help what the psyche has instructed the will.

It resembles a spouse guaranteeing her significant other that what he has chosen is correct. At the point when we have an opposite image of a couple — the spouse concluding everything and the husband coming in just as a "yes" man — then we likewise obtain a converse outcome.

Insight is intended to find out accuracy. The psyche is the able organ for seeing. Insight can be sharpened to such sharpness and precision that reality becomes planer to see. At the point when you understand the situation of a circumstance with your brain, and provide the psyche with complete order, you are better prepared to answer.

Ace your emotions

There are times when you have a precise impression of an improvement, however at that point the Emotions freely settle on an alternate course. The will, at a loss regarding where to go (there are times when you are "unsure" about something), would grip to the more grounded force, which is either the brain or the Emotions . On the off chance that this is consistently the situation, you see a hesitant individual generally uncertain about things. He is handily conflicted between an impulse and an idea.

The psyche plainly should manage over emotion and will. There ought to be no split difference in this. Achievement really relies on how enabled the psyche is.

The psyche is prepared to lead through day-to-day straightforward activities that increase as progress goes on. It is customised to order and be complied by the Emotions by advising the will to agree with its position against a pessimistic inclination or the other way around. The psyche can likewise advise the Emotions to agree with its position against an obstinate will.

In basic activities, the psyche is prepared to expect a telling mode. The acquiescence of the Emotions and will builds up this. A win is modified for the brain and the activity's expansion in level and power. This is more than once finished over a significant stretch until the course of the brain telling the Emotions and will become programmed and momentary.

At the point when the brain has dominated the directing mode, it is exposed to a more elevated level and prepared to order the Emotions as well as the entire body. Indeed, even the deliberate frameworks and cycles in the body are endeavoured to be directed for positive outcomes.

Ace your emotions

As the brain advances and is given more power, it is then moved into a higher component of force — the ability to order things outside the body.

Notice the contemplations you have during the day. Where does your psyche meander to when you are driving, strolling, or your hands are occupied? **What sort of inside exchange do you have when you are confronted with difficulties, negative circumstances, or the everyday parts of day-to-day existence?**

Assuming your responses to those questions were connected with negative idea examples or propensities, begin to supplant them with positive ones.

Begin by recognizing the pieces of your life that will generally cause pessimistic sentiments and contemplations. It very well may be a relationship, your regularly scheduled drive, colleagues, a relative, workplace, or other obligations.

Then, at that point, consider positive ways you can move toward these conditions. Begin little by zeroing in on each issue in turn and apply standards of positive brain research with self-talk and a decent mentality.

Emotions are most likely not a declaration of general encounters. Surely, numerous theoreticians expect a collection of Emotions that are normal for all individuals, with respect to model, dread, outrage, distress, satisfaction, shock and revulsion. A portion of these responses is normal to a few different warm-blooded creatures as well as people. A few Emotions can be evoked naturally. furthermore, what brings out them can likewise be unique. The judgment of various Emotions ' worth is moreover not the equivalent 100% of the time. Emotions are attached to normal natural circumstances, yet in addition to changing social circumstances. Martha

Nussbaum claims in Disturbances of Thought. The Mental fortitude of Emotions that "people experience Emotions in manners that are formed both by individual history and by normal practices". She figures that Emotions are "... components of our normal animality with extensive versatile importance: so their natural premise is probably going to be normal to all".But she rapidly adds, "However this doesn't imply that Emotions are not contrastingly moulded by various social orders". She calls attention to a few wellsprings of social variety herself. In any case, states of assuming a significant part. In addition to other things various social orders are defenceless against various sorts of chance, something that normally has significance for encounters of dread, for instance. Furthermore, mystical, strict and cosmological conviction frameworks impact our profound encountered.